PARKINSON'S

Day by Day

by

Ed Kluft

With special contributions by

Sheila Feige

Kluft Publishing

ISBN-13: 978-1517189419 // ISBN-10: 1517189411

Kluft Publishing
The Villages, Florida

TABLE OF CONTENTS

ED 1

SHEILA 51

CARE GIVERS 127

DEDICATION

Forever we remember these family members and their profound influence on our lives.

Son ~ Phillip

Dad ~ Nathan

Mom ~ Dorothy

Edward Boorstein

Stanley Snyder

The friends we miss:
Sam Wool

Edward Stoll

Barry DePristo

FROM THE AUTHORS

This is not an exclusive experience. It is what we all go through, or will, after contracting The Disease. We've written this from anger and in progression. Some names have been omitted to protect those who want their problem kept private.

A special thanks for the originators of the exercise format we call "The Parkinson's Fight Club".

Also, a special thanks to Ed's son and sister, her husband and Sheila's husband and family. By our writing this, they now understand better what we and others like us cannot avoid enduring.

What we do know is that we don't know. We can only hope to live long enough to make a difference.

Book #1

For Men

PARKINSON'S

as experienced

Day by Day

Ed Kluft

ED

This is not an exclusive experience ... it is what we all experience or will, as anyone will, after contracting The Disease. I've written this from anger and in progression as the disease has progressed. If it is repetitious, it is because Parkinson's itself is repetitious—painfully, maddeningly repetitious. I have omitted names for those who want their problem kept private. Others have given permission for me to include their names.

I was diagnosed approximately seven years ago; I was 72 years old. Terrible day to find out I had Parkinson's disease (PD). Parkinson's is the general term for those symptoms that can give a clue to the problems to follow or those already experienced. It can also be a false indication that I have the disease.

A diagnosis could be MS or Muscular Dystrophy or even dementia. Each person has different symptoms as a rule even if it is PD. The General Rule is once diagnosed add five years to it; I believe more.

I was having a problem where my walking pace became a shuffle. It was a short pace I hadn't noticed. At the same time I was having a problem getting out of a chair and my bed. First, after I moved to Florida I noticed my bowling game had drastically deteriorated. I left Connecticut with my third relationship, Phillis, and a 170 average and then I found my brain wouldn't tell my hand where to send the ten pin ball. After two years in our community league with this problem, I retired my game. Knowing I had a coordination problem I decided to take several months with a trainer at The Villages Wellness Center after work three evenings a week. With the assistance of the trainer I worked on the varied machines she thought were best for me. I improved my power and trimmed down in weight. I looked good but still had my problems getting off a gurney and on and off the medicine ball. It was scary because of my balance problem and that was all too new to me. She thought it was good training for me. No. I never could get comfortable. I couldn't keep it from rolling sideways and backwards even with her steadying the large ball. The clincher came next when I had to walk on a 3″ wide black painted stripe on the floor. I was too unsteady to make it 20 feet without stepping off more than once. That line was a sure sign that I had a serious problem.

We want to deny having a problem. Boy, I was wrong. I could no longer deny that I now had a shuffle, tremors in my left hand and was very unsteady with my balance. Luckily I had never fallen, which is a common problem with most PD victims.

Almost immediately I made an appointment with a neurologist in The Villages, my home community in Florida. Typically, Phillis and I waited before being shown into the examining room to wait 15 or 20 minutes more for the doctor. Finally the door opened and the doctor standing there ten feet away looked across the room at me sitting next to Phillis and said, "You have Parkinson's". How the hell did he give a diagnosis without an exam? He said, I had the Parkinson's mask. I showed no facial expression as I looked at him. He went on to prove his point by tapping my forehead just a little above my eyes and said, "Don't blink." I said that it's not possible to make a judgment just with that test. He did it several more times and I couldn't stop blinking. Until he did it to Phillis and I saw she didn't blink I became somewhat of a believer. Following that, he made an appointment to have an MRI which subsequently proved I had the disease.

Now that we knew the worst was true, the doctor made an appointment at the hospital to test me for a new breakthrough called DBS. Deep Brain Stimulation would alter the brain and the unwanted motions I had. After two days of tests for the surgery I got devastating news: I did not qualify. When I went home with the bad news, I asked Phillis if we were to get rid of one of our two cars, which she would choose. Her natural question was, "Why?" The answer I gave was because I was going to smash it—and me—into a tree. My symptoms didn't match their chart. Wow, now where do I go from here? As it turned out, DBS has proven to be a failure in most cases. Some getting the treatment have had an adverse reaction. I was given a prescription for Dopamine, not the name of the medication but a neurotransmitter which my brain was not producing in the quantity that it required. The doses prescribed made me feel a little better but I still had those telltale signs of the disease—the shuffle, the tremors, the lack of balance. I could not deny them any longer!

I still couldn't get out of a chair at home and especially in restaurants. Getting out of a chair I required someone to extend a hand or arm for me to pull myself up. Luckily I had never fallen, which is a common problem with most PD victims.

*****

Special note: (January, 2015) Just approved for testing wearing a small computer that will administer dopamine in small amounts regularly to the small intestines. If successful, it will make me feel better almost immediately.

*****

I'd had this problem for more than two years at this point. I can remember school days in D.C. where my balance was a problem, but not so that I couldn't play tennis and swim in AAU races, often to a winning finish. I think to myself, *would I ever be able to deal with this horrific feeling that I had been losing my hearing even before being diagnosed?* If it weren't for arguing with some frequency with my house mate (we are not married), I would have lost the sound totally as so many PD victims have. PD robs the victim of speech volume, but the voice can be regained with proper training. Another side effect of the disease is getting anger when told something more than once. My memory has been getting worse. This *could* be my age, which would be somewhat normal. But it could be Parkinson's.

Before the disease I became an entrepreneur after two years of accounting school. Furniture was my family's business and I followed suit. In 1970 I opened my first furniture store. I worked and worried seven days and nights a week, devoting little time to reading anything but trade papers and the local newspapers. I played tennis, golf and water skied in the few hours I allowed myself once the kids were old enough. I performed in those sports well enough that I felt socially acceptable. I had some close friends from school who would tolerate my odd schedule. Most close ties were one at a time. Except for my closest friend, who was 50 when his lungs gave out and died, I am still in touch with the others. As of this update, the two others have passed, one three years ago and the final of my closest died four weeks ago. I'm 79 and there's no one to corroborate my stories as I remember them. I feel slightly alone at this time, July, 2014.

I probably experienced the first symptoms

of the disease thirty years ago when riding horses in Arizona and in the Poconos. I rode often each year though the symptoms didn't bother me during those times. I didn't think of them as symptoms then. There's no evidence of a time table of when symptoms begin nor is PD known to be hereditary. What we do know is that we don't know. Our *Daily Sun* newspaper ran an article on DBS twice, the Deep Brain Stimulation, and I was offended and so disappointed because those of us that could did not qualify were never mentioned.

I wrote my anger to the *Daily Sun* "Letters To the Editor" stating that they failed to mention those of us who are the victims of Parkinson's and for whom DBS holds no promise.. It read: "Operation is not the only option for Parkinson's victims. I was diagnosed six years ago and had the typical pattern of walking in small shuffling steps and tremors on my left side along with other symptoms normally associated with the disease. I could not turn without fearing I would lose my balance. I feared backing up to a wall and not knowing where it would be. I explained how I trained myself to not show the Parkinsonism's we call the appearance that tell we have the disease". I went on to describe what I go through to avoid what I had to deal with in the Parkinson's life that I know now. The article was a great success, I got a call from the leader of what's known as The Fight Club to come to their support group and tell my story. I got several other calls from people who wanted more information. I continued to go to the group to exercise. In these past five years it has grown from 30 to 120 in season attending three times a week. Half of those coming are care givers who participate in the exercising for their own health.

Many of us had the new Logo with two red boxing gloves embroidered on some of our shirts. I'm proud to wear these shirts. The mission is to have us fight this dreaded disease through exercise in tempo to music. Since there is no cure, the intent is to hold the disease to a tolerable level through a process the leader feels will help him improve as we do. He has had his fight 15 years. His energy is now so great I can only hope to get mine to his level. It's so great that we are entertained just trying to go through the motions with him. There have been some that have complained about his energy. They just don't like it. I say, "Poo poo on them." They can't see the socializing aspect of his exercise sessions. At least those few are communicating, the important aspect of holding Parkinson's at bay. SECs—they need more 'sex' in their life. Our creed was we must SOCIALIZE, EXERSIZE, and COMMUNICATE abbreviated to … (SEX) every day thirty minutes for survival.

Getting out of bed continues to be a problem. It is still very difficult. My muscle tone is not adequate. Fortunately the night stand next to me is heavy and rigid enough for me to grab the edge to pull myself up after swinging my legs over the side of the bed. Then to make it out of the bedroom or into the bathroom, I have to have a hand on the furniture each step on the way. From there I would hold on to the door jams which I still must do five years later. I don't want to risk falling and hurting myself as so many continue to do once the problem begins. Again, my muscle toning was not adequate. To be exact I required muscle retraining. I did it. I reeducated my brain, as I thought, by taking charge. The neurologist said he had not seen it accomplished by other patients. I had two, three people a week come up to me to say they've been watching and they have not seen any signs of Parkinson's. Believe me, as I'm writing this I feel the motion inside my system and know I still have the dreaded Parkinson's disease. I don't know how or where it will progress before a cure is in.

I have returned to the neurologist who sent me to the MRI and now he feels I might possibly have Mèniére's disease causing the hissing sound I have in my ears. He prescribed two medications to deal with my inner ear that might relate to dizziness. I don't know if I'll ever feel better in my present state of mind. These are two new meds that should prevent seasickness and certainly have me spend a lot of time peeing. I spent five days on the two meds and I have gotten severely unstable and have abdominal pain at night. I stopped both tablets until I was to see him the following week.

I was scheduled to have vertigo therapy. My mental and physical feelings have become so severe that I was going to admit myself to the Hospital. I drove myself safely but decided the hospital could not do more than my two doctors have done. I stopped for breakfast. I don't want go to a hospital since I've heard from several people saying they won't give me my Parkinson's pills on my schedule. They said the staff would not only discourage me from taking my own meds but would administer pills only on their rounds. August 2, I was given three more tests by the neurologist. Test 1—an hour and half spent measuring my brain activity. Tests 2 & 3, for balance, were somewhat repetitious. I had already investigated vertigo. No new information came out of those tests.

Early May, 2013, a year after I started putting these memories on paper, new experiences keep popping up. Sometime earlier that year I had begun to experience dyskinesia, starting with my head and continuing down through my shoulders to my waist. It manifests itself with an uncontrollable weaving motion mostly from left to right and with accompanied head bobbing.

Suddenly on **Monday, May 21st**, after morning exercise, I went to our den and stood at my computer armoire. Standing there I began my first severe dizzy attack. WOW ... just standing was impossible. I chose to fall back into my recliner just behind me and there it got worse. It felt like the recliner was turning over with me in it. I thought, *I'm dying, I'm going to hit the floor, it's a stroke and I'm going to vomit.* I screamed, "Phillis! Phillis!" and she called from the phone, "What do you want?" When she finally came into the den, she said "Don't scream, but say please come to me." At that time I needed support immediately. I didn't feel anything but panic fear and need. I didn't have time to be polite.

Today, still in **May, 2013**, Phillis left for Connecticut and left me with the two dogs. I had put my name in to play golf Tuesday morning but called to cancel. I felt somewhat dizzy. I don't know what will happen if I have a fall and no one is here to help or take the dogs, should it be necessary. I have the instruction of what to do for the vertigo in form of exercise which I can do between one portion at home and the other at our Wellness Center nearby. I really don't know why, but too many of us PDs are having the same experiences. We see each other deteriorating as time goes on. We exercise regularly to slow the process down but it's a progressive disease without an end in sight. I have to remind myself that to continue to live life with Parkinson's disease you have just to "fight, fight, fight". I try. Every day now I have some period where I am truly sick. It's not the dizziness but a nauseous feeling that throwing up would help. If I could purge the feeling, I think it would be a relief. It's hateful, but I keep on going or least I think I'm dealing with it.

Nothing more until the following **Tuesday, May 28** after 9 holes of golf, finishing and getting home at 10AM. I was feeling O.K. I took the two little Yorkies to the park where they relieved themselves and did some running. This is a morning routine for me. While standing that morning in the field, that dizzy feeling returned. Aware of the danger, I tried to stand still with nothing to hold on to see if it would pass. I knew to get close to the ground to prevent a fall that might hurt. The feeling this time told me I would fall sideways, but no, I could not stop myself from falling backwards to the ground. A lady and gentleman came quickly to help me up. I had fallen for the third time in two weeks. I had felt that I was in control of the disease and its symptoms. I knew that day that I was getting worse despite seeing two doctors, my family doctor and my neurologist.

We have a reprint from the newspaper. The leader and originator of our group is in wearing his white hat which he never is seen without even in public. I'm always in no hat, no hair. He has taught us drumming as one of our exercises. Without exception, the neurologist who has visited with us has been simply amazed how we have learned the drumming routine. Every PD person has been able to enjoy this exercise. We drum at the start of each session then he talks about the disease and even how it's affected his life.

Morning is a night. I get up between 4 and 5 each morning and go to my computer after taking the dogs out. Sometime around mid-day to late afternoon it's *yuck* again. We're frequently asked when our up times and down times happen each day. I can't pin that time down for a regular pattern. I can say that as I write this entry I am getting worse. Since waking up this morning, I have been very unsteady and that ill feeling is still with me. In addition something is new: my left hip hurts when I move. It has become terribly painful when I get up or down. I am walking full time on a cane. I am stopping my twice-a-week vertigo treatment mostly because the $50 or $75 co-pay is too much for my budget. I haven't fallen in a couple weeks; I still feel I could have a severe attack. I'm now very depressed over my condition.

Contrary to my normal pattern, I awoke this morning feeling much better. I have no answers for the why or how I might feel from day to day. My depression is gone and this being Saturday I will be bowling this morning. My hip problem has lessened. I don't question the why any more. It is a day by day life now. However, now its 10:30AM and I'm back home after quitting bowling by myself. Midway through our session, I became dizzy and nauseous. So much for my beginning a good day.

I have sent this page to Phillis to share with her family up north if she chooses to. In three more days she'll be back here in Florida. I don't want to be a burden on her. I cannot stop being short-tempered. I'm doing the best I can. This disease makes us prone to impatience and to allow our tempers to act up. I don't know if she will ever show this rant of mine to her daughters; I will in time. Until there's a preventive measure, one or more of her four daughters and their husbands might develop MS or more likely Parkinson's. I'd like to say life goes on but with this disease every day is a chore.

As I am constantly aware, these diseases are in my body and do not necessarily show in my demeanor. I try not to show I have any of them. My memory is pitiful. That's the dementia which I kiddingly say started in the third grade. I was never a good student. I made it through, however, always in the bottom half of my class. Having all these diseases working individually or sometime together is exhausting. They are all so deep that hiding what's happening is very tiring, especially the dyskinesia, if I'm aware of it. But right now I'm mostly concerned about the dementia. It's a little known fact that 75% to 80% of Parkinson sufferers will develop dementia which will develop into Alzheimer's. That's when we all start our last journey. What a disgusting way to put it.

There have been upward of forty-eight deaths in the past five years in this community, some too early and some not so bad. A terrible reality all learn to accept. We don't know when however. We all ask each other how we're doing only to hear, "Not so well." Another question, have you fallen lately? It seems someone has an arm in a sling or others have bruises. I have been lucky, no pains from falls yet but maybe bouncing off walls. Not pleasant. Only now I'm having a problem with the return of a shuffle when I turn in a small area. It's exhausting and difficult to be mobile without my cane. I suspect it to be my dosage or mixture of the meds.

My neurologist had no thoughts to offer outside of walk down the hall turn and come back and see me in February which is six months, typical. There's no help on the way; I don't look for flashing red lights rushing to rescue me. The best is to talk to other PD sufferers to see what they're doing. They have their own problems and without answers they are experiencing a slow deterioration as I do. Although there are those of us that for some reason do a rapid nosedive and suddenly they are gone. The constant reminder: Parkinson's = progressive, degenerative.

My family has praised these notes which I send as updates. My loving son says he tears when reading them. I have had my years and hope they won't have the same experiences. It is as we know it to be, more prevalent for this disease to attack an older group, people in their sixties and up. MS, which is similar in reaction, is more commonly attacking at a younger age, the teens and up. We have a few people with MS who come exercise with us. We have a stroke victim exercising with us. His support group doesn't exercise; they talk to inform. Talk helps in understanding, but without muscle toning as well as learning to maintain your vocal cords to prevent losing the ability to talk, we lose ground faster necessary. We all need our speech to communicate. As our throat begins to close eating becomes more difficult. This can signify the beginning of the end. We *must* keep our vocal cords working!

This morning I was very unsteady once out of bed. Why? You tell me. I wasn't bouncing off the walls, though my legs felt like jelly. Now two mornings later, I was wakened by a vertigo dizzy attack. I feared getting out of bed, I wasn't feeling safe getting up, I took a vertigo pill and it had no effect. I had a piece of toast all in the hope that it might be a problem with my stomach. An hour and half later I took my four morning pills which included the vertigo tablet again. Why, since the feeling is so overwhelming, am I able to write this paragraph without falling off my desk chair? Don't answer; there isn't an answer to why on any of this. I made it through October still feeling a bit woozy most of the days. Making turns and starting to walk forward I'm doing small shuffle steps which is debilitating.

I was a Poster Boy in eliminating the shuffle. So now what? I'll put a shroud over the poster if I see it. There is no promise of a better life. I have to want to deal with these changes even knowing I will never improve permanently. My new acquaintances over these past few years and I agree that this is for the shits. Without exception, we are all sinking at the same pace. We bear the best we can and will continue to do so. A respected acquaintance, an

American and former officer in the Israeli army died today. He did a sudden down turn proving we don't die from Parkinson's itself but one of the medical problems under the Parkinson Umbrella. I had a retched day yesterday feeling sick to my stomach and very weak on my legs. I continue to use my cane full time in and out of the house now. I do have a Walker but I seldom use it. The stores we frequent like the drug stores and grocery stores have their carts for me to hang onto. I use it where I shouldn't be, the casino. One of my med's side-effects says—*gambling*.

This is the end of October and the disease is taking over my life. I sleep comfortably but fear how I feel getting out of bed. The Parkinson shuffle is back and my legs feel painful. I don't want to and haven't fallen lately. I will. What do I do? Where do I retreat now that I see my body strength slipping away? At this point life is not promising. I'm going to need help and I fear no one would want to be my care-giver. Of some fifty care givers in our group, each has complained of what is expected of them. With all this going on, I'm still expected to do general housework both in and around the house. I just don't feel I'm able to fulfill the list that has been given to me. Worse, I'm given reminders all day, every day, of what is on my work list.

One of the most pronounced problems of our disease is being told anything repeatedly. I certainly have that going on. I feel, Help, Help, but no help coming. This is another problem day starting. Please give me the strength and humor I need. I said much earlier in this tale, dying is the best way out. I don't believe in a life after, but if there is, I have a son and dad I'd like to see.

Today, Wednesday, I go to exercise at noon and then I bowl from 3 to 5. My game has not been the game I had in Connecticut. It is exercise both Wednesdays and Saturday mornings. Every day I have what I call very sick times and then it seems they pass. This turn to the worse seems to coincide with the first day with vertigo. There seems to be hope, several people have said they had it and with the help of the same meds which I take their vertigo has gone away. So? I'm waiting.

October 25, 2013, I am suffering terribly with the feeling of nausea, weakening in my legs and my brain spitting out commands to shuffle again. Earlier I talked how I felt in control of my body movements. I have totally lost that and feel helpless. I wonder if mixing the vertigo med with the others I take could be the problem. Doctors are not able to provide the answers as we wish they would. There are no answers and I have no direction to solve this terrible world I'm forced to live in. Hospital or assisted living is definitely not the answer. Three days now and I am experiencing a very large increase in my feeling I might fall. I haven't fallen yet but I have ended the experiment in cutting back the doses of medication that I thought might have been the cause in my downturn. **Day 4**, I have returned to my regular prescribed dosages and feel slight improvement. So much for my experimentation for now. I'm having anxiety attacks. I have to find somewhere else where I can stay, a place where I can have some peace with fewer verbal confrontations.

November 6, **Wednesday,** I have an appointment with my primary doctor. I've been told that a seasick pill might work better for my vertigo. Just to prove everyone has an opinion. I'll check back here with a report. The doctor said a pill like Dramamine reacts when motion such as flying or boating is not what I'm looking for. His recommendation is to stop the pill I'm on until I feel an attack coming. Funny how seeing a doctor works. I felt better and tested much better in his office. Confirmed, see your doctor to cure problems by themselves. Meanwhile I'm off the vertigo pill and have felt considerably better. I hate to get back to normal when I can feel ill and complain to someone. My only fear is I might live longer. I still will always have the "Parkinsonism diseases" in me.

This week forty-two people including their care givers (their spouses) went on an annual cruse in the Caribbean and I being a social person was left behind. The way I was feeling I thought it would be best. I was appointed as the substitute for Monday exercise leader. Except for our leader and his dynamic energy we did well. Not easy but as the apt manager I chose a few others to do most of what I was instructed to do. Monday mornings are men only days with donuts. I picked them up. I was told by several that I did a great job. I asked myself what the hell I did outside of organizing the function. We exercise to music after we do the drumming exercises we've learned. Drumming is very unusual but we understand the necessity in doing what our brains need—using left and right hands as we drum. Our leader has been all across the country attending support group sessions including the several that are right here in Florida. Other groups seem to discuss the problems we have with the disease but do no exercise. Without the exercise we lose muscle tone. This much we know. After 30 minutes we've done well. Every day we exercise ten minutes three times at home to music. It works. It lessens Parkinson's symptoms. We each feel a little better after exercising.

In the past five years, and without my really knowing, some thirty-eight people just from our group have died. Several are in the final stages bedding down in assisted living and rehab centers without the ability to manage the life that Parkinson's has dealt them. I must say again, losing movement control, inability to swallow and diminished voice volume are the signs. We have known cases of some who have given up and stopped drinking and eating to end their misery. I have just visited a good acquaintance who is in a rehab center. He looked wrinkled, gaunt and pale and in addition, he could hardly talk. He's there because of several falling episodes. Stories like his become quite common. I dread to think how I might go. Can we sink that low and come back to a reasonable life? Not usually. We talk openly among ourselves about how we're each deteriorating and how our deaths will eventually come. Personally, there are dreadful times that death would be welcomed. I go to my family doctor who's happy to watch my health. I shy away from my neurologist at least until they have some answers. A while back in this memoir I listed seven diseases I have in my system. Only my strength and determination will allow me to survive. Exercise is the key to delaying the obvious. *I don't love exercising but it is a must for survival.*

A new chapter: No question. PARKINSON'S IS THE DAWNING OF A NEW LIFE. What I was rarely thinking about, my old life has been replaced by totally new challenges without room to reminisce about what was. This is worse than when I was diagnosed. I am light-headed and feel that I could be dizzy and fall or weakened legs could cause me to fall. I did go back to play golf yesterday after a three month layoff but I didn't feel comfortable enough to go past the 8th hole. My legs were weakening. I will try bowling after we exercise this afternoon. If that fails I will have a dim future. I must regain my strength and exercising is the only way back. Writing this memoir has helped in giving me a reason to exist. Sounds harsh, but it is what keeps my mind going. Our brain controls everything we do and keeping the mind active is the best exercise, thereby slowing the start of dementia. Last evening I played three handed Gin Rummy and it makes me *think* and that strategy is brain strengthening. Changing a light bulb is not as useful.

This awful feeling! My stomach hurts, my dyskinesia is exhausting and trying not to fall adds to my dissatisfaction with this new life. I'm fighting to get back to a normal strut without the recurring shuffle. I keep repeating to myself, *I want the normal life back that I lost three weeks ago.* Sleeping is a challenge when I get as little four and a half hours and when I seldom get seven to eight hours. I still feel it's not enough. I took myself off the vertigo med I think could have triggered the new discomfort. Every med is a trial to see if it works with those I am already taking. Sad, but the doctors don't know what to prescribe next. There has not been a breakthrough in the years since my diagnosis even with the mega-funds Michael J. Fox has put into research. It seems that research for cancer has made more progress recently.

Three days ago I was able to walk, no cane, no shuffle and no tremors. I thought more normalcy had returned. As usual I was wrong. I went bowling and played 9 holes of golf then wasn't comfortable in the days that followed. We're at the end of November and I feel the same and wish the manageable feeling would return.

I have to laugh. The other evening I drank a scotch and water and it nearly knocked me off my feet. I knew it would not go with one of my meds. The same thing happened a couple times this past year. If you don't mind a little sarcasm, I'm elated that I have to cut out a social drink with friends and cut way back on my habit for sugar products. I will find out which meds are giving me this problem and maybe I can become a little more social. I have never been in any need of alcohol except in a social atmosphere.

As the days and the problems continue onward I now have fear of losing my balance. Just this morning, **Saturday, 23rd of November**, I was so dazed in getting out of bed that falling seemed eminent. I moved slowly hanging on to furniture and door jams to prevent my falling, of course. This is the deterioration of my better health. The same is happening to many of our friends in our support group. Can I reverse this trend? I don't know. Our exercise guru talks about his own problems but still remains very agile. He runs, walks eight miles every morning before dawn. He is an inspiration to all of us. The **following Monday** was probably the worst I've had in a year. I felt ill all day, unsteady and very unsocial. All of this is not new in this writing but writing keeps my mind in better condition. I thank those of you who are reading this for your help. Knowing others will read it helps tremendously.

What the hell is this bizarre disease doing? It's nuts. When the inevitable question comes up at exercise, "What is your up or down time each day?" my answer varies. I'd like to answer but can't. This morning I woke up weaker than usual. Ugh. I won't give up but I still feel I can prevent falling. At noon I went to our group health exercise program and following that tedium I went bowling. It's not something that gets rave notice, but I do feel good about the

accomplishment. However, after playing golf
and bowling, I have a downturn that makes
turning and walking without a cane next to
impossible. As much as I can recall every day
has the same pattern. I haven't narrowed it
down to what time of day the down period
might be. There has to be a better way to go
after all. We don't even know where this one
came from. I'm the only one ever in our family
that has had this much 'fun'.

While the days bump along, I continue to
wake up. That's the good news. Right now I'm
weak in the legs and slightly unbalanced. I did
ten minutes exercising to the music from The
Villages weather station. It's a good tempo
usually in the old rock music. I finished and
moved to my computer so I could tell you. I'll
do the same mid-day. We do have up times and
down times. Tell me when my up time is so I
can enjoy a short bit of it. It varies and doesn't
last long. Gee ... this new life is a trip, full of
laughter like, ha ha. In the beginning the
symptoms were hardly noticeable until finally I
did notice while in the hands of a pretty

German trainer. However, she didn't suggest I might have something more than a coordination problem that creeps up in our senior years. At that time I was seventy years old. I had Parkinson's and worked very hard in getting rid of the appearance of Parkinson's and the normal tremor that I had on my left. I didn't know I was walking with small shuffling steps. Learning how to retrain these problems and look very normal worked. This is written 5 years later and once again I have a problem with the shuffle but no tremors. I'm so conscious of a brain malfunction it leaves me in search of why it came back. There were only two of us in a sixty support group that had no signs of the "Parkinsonisms" which are the signs of the disease. Now I'm on a cane and walker when necessary. Hence, The Dawning of a New Life.

Am I repeating myself? Well, yes. Parkinson's is repetitive. It just repeats symptoms with no warning and no reason. I never had good coordination and now, like rubbing your stomach while patting your head moving to the tempo of music seems to help. My arms have to go one way or another while at the same time my legs have to work in other directions. Then there's the direction my upper body ought to go. My coordination, or lack of it, gets in my way.

I'm having punk days now. Funny, when this first happened, I considered ending my life. That was the last I was depressed and I feel differently since I started telling this story. It has given meaning to my existence to get to the computer to tell you how terrible this disease can be. It's like driving a horse-drawn carriage shouting, "This stinks! How many would you like?"

Vertigo raises questions. Is there a specific trigger like a certain food? I have not been able to discover one food that I think is culprit. The slightest bit of alcohol is out indefinitely. One sip of beer last night gave me a vertigo spin that was devastating but I didn't fall to the floor. My housemate caught me as I was falling off the counter stool. I really would like to write in a more entertaining way but those of you that are experiencing the disease will relate to these events. I look forward to going to sleep for four to five hours of peace. When I get up I first test to see if my sea legs are intact. Then it's up to me to change my diet habits to be super cautious once I'm up. **Three days before Christmas, 2013**, and I played what I feel was the final round of golf. My legs would not hold up and I quit on the 4th hole. I'll try to get back as soon as my strength returns. Since that time it has been touch and go whether my legs would cooperate. One more time and I had to quit playing for a while. Haven't played since the first of the year.

It's now six month later, **June, 2014,** and the telltale problem is back. I look more like I have Parkinson's after I'd been so successful hiding the signs for at least three years. The past three days I have been feeling more ill than I can tolerate. I feel sick and can't describe what the feeling is. My legs ache, which saps my energy. Thank goodness for this book. It helps me focus on something other than the pain.

I have convinced a good lady friend to

write her twenty-year experience with PD. She is now a co-author of this book, Sheila Feige. I find her the most interesting feisty person to work with.

My writing and Sheila's together are for the benefit of perhaps you or someone you know who has these same problems. Failing to recognize these signs can be fatal. There are many out in our area as you may guess that choose to stay in their homes to hide what they know and won't show it. We've done everything we can to get them in to what we call "The Parkinson Exercise Club". Again, we talk about those who are hiding and our not being able coax them out to our support group. They are committing themselves to a speedier death. Yes, we use the word "death" freely because it is the reason for our road coming to an end all too quickly when exercise can prolong the inevitable.

This is **July 15, 2014**, and it is the day I felt better and walked more normally. It's been a week of horror when not waking in the morning would have been a blessing. Walking with a shuffle, headachy and less vision. Still can't figure when and how many pills to take to get back on track. I saw a new urologist today and my PSA was way too high. "Might be cancerous, come back in 6 months and retest." I told him, a very nice young doctor, that I will not elect any surgery or treatment if I do have a malignancy. He understood I would ride it out to the end. I've been very satisfied with my life and accomplishments.

My PD coach and co-author, Sheila, has experienced the progression of cancer with another person some years ago. I wasn't going to pursue the testing much further but with her insistence I will be pursuing the potential problem now. The first test is for the Prostrate and that will be **August 7, 2014**. Unfortunately it is a Thursday and I will miss an exercise session. Gary, Sheila's husband will drive me. I'm not allowed to drive under the influence of a 'mild dose of something to relax' me.

July18, my handwriting and printing has gotten more unsteady. Doing display and design has been most enjoyable and creative for me in my businesses. It's slipping away as those ahead of me have experienced. Thank goodness for the computer.

I'm jumping in again to tell you how bad the past few days have been, and then how, like a prayer come true, I got up feeling steady on my feet and feeling like I might survive this. The start of the difficult time I believe was an MSG, Monosodium Glutamate, attack; in this case from eating crispy fried chicken with the seasoning. In the down times my legs become painfully weak. I do really have to do leg exercises to increase my stamina. I started going to a Thursday exercise group for two hours. It is more of a balance program unlike the movement to tempo of the other group. I am still disappointed that the "Parkinsonisms" are back and so evident. I have the small shuffle as I start to step and same as I turn in a small area. I have to get back to MOM, "mind over matter". It seems I watch good friends gradually deteriorating each week. I have to increase my exercise time to postpone my own deterioration. I have started doing full leg bends ten at a time. Then my legs hurt from stiffness after doing the bends and I have to walk the stiffness off.

A word about support groups: The previous Thursday group had a split for a reason no one seems to remember or want to tell. Out of that group came the Parkinson's Fight Club©. Meeting on Wednesdays, Sundays and Men Only on Mondays early with coffee and donuts. On the Mondays Men Only discussions would be what women would not contribute to. Out of that time the Women, mostly all Care givers, are meeting for breakfast after dropping the men at their Monday meeting. It's good for them to share their experiences. I've gotten vital information from them for this book.

I found last Thanksgiving that I couldn't drink anything with alcohol, not even beer or wine. I believe it didn't mix with one of my meds. I'm off the Dramamine now and I would really like to try a little Red Wine. I hope the issue is a non-issue now. I'd so like to go out and have a drink as I used to with people and feel a little more social. This damned disease has put a damper on my social life. Sitting quietly aside listening is more my speed now. I have decided to find some social groups for me to socialize with and be more engaging. Of course, I have to remember I have Parkinson's and have people around that will be tolerant when necessary.

I had a friend with PD who could commiserate about the anxieties of displaying "Parkinsonisms" at a party. I do miss that comfort. I'm not happy about the prospect of giving up driving. The time hasn't come yet! I'll be able to continue driving in The Villages. Do I have choices at that stage of my life? Perhaps not. That's a bridge I'll have to cross later. Right now the Parkinson's group is my family. In this time period, as my symptoms have worsened, I have to ask, "What can I do, increase my dosage or decrease them?" Again, there is no doctor who can answer the question definitely. I'll do a series of experiments on my own. Doesn't seem a logical way, but my guess is as good as theirs I've learned.

The past two or three days have been a horror. My legs have been hurting and I've been frightened that I will lose my balance and fall. Fortunately I haven't. Two days ago, Saturday, we had my step-daughter, her husband and his mother, all from Connecticut, visit for the day. They were enjoyable, we went to lunch at one of our favorite restaurants on the very large Little Lake Weir, Gator Joes. The restaurant has a beach on one side mostly with teeny boppers in skimpy bikinis and on the other side small boats tied up or anchored in shallow water. We sat outside in 80 degrees, a mild breeze and bright sunshine. Despite the atmosphere I wasn't feeling really well. I should love my Parkinson's, it's the life I live with. That was Saturday.

On Sunday I had dinner with a neighbor who lives up our block. Corned beef and cabbage—delicious! My birthday, you know.

I was born on St. Paddy's Day in 1936. What a glorious day. I was there though I don't remember any of it, of course. What is interesting though is that I do remember being in my crib. I was in long enough to stand at the lift rail. This silly subject reminds me of being back in Connecticut in my furniture store where a customer came in to shop for a bed for her daughter who had outgrown the length of her crib. The daughter must have been five or six years old. It took the woman three more trips in to get up the nerve to make the purchase of a standard twin bed. She was so afraid that her daughter would fall out of a big girl bed. We added guardrails to prevent the child from falling off the bed.

One odder story in the hundreds that could be told was the young couple shopping for a three-piece bedroom group: bed, chest and night table. They came to a decision and we went to the counter where I wrote the sale and gave them the total amount due. The young man said abruptly, "Wait. We want to talk about the price." My reply was that we had talked about the price already, hadn't we? "Well yes, but my dad said never pay the first quote." Again, as the owner of the store and feeling strongly in charge, I asked if they had shopped up and down the street and he said they had. I asked if we were the best quality and best price, which I knew, he said we were. Well? They couldn't buy, dad won out and they left. They never came back. Hell, I could have given them a lamp for the night stand. It would have cost me so little to clinch the sale. But I was on my last weekend because I had sold the store. I didn't lose anything and would not have gained anything for me personally. I turned the keys over to the new owner and continued as a factory rep. After a year I moved to Florida and took over that territory.

The irony is a year later the buyer of my store went bankrupt and that payment stopped. Not too long after that disappointment, the two factories I sold for also went out of business. I applied for a sales position at a retail store and after two years there they went out also. Boy, I'm now very retired. These failures were a result of the devastation in the early 2000s. I had nineteen furniture store accounts of which only four remained in business. The cost in traveling had gone up so that I couldn't continue being a factory representative. Funny how these memories pop up. But it's good to remember the good days when I ran a successful business regardless of what happened to it—and me— afterwards.

It's now **April 24, 2014** and my legs are getting more difficult to manage because of two factors, one being a general weakness and the other the Parkinson's brain not processing my coordination. This causes my feet to shudder in a sense before I can stretch my steps out to a normal pace. Just today my health insurance carrier called to give me a location nearby to exercise as frequently as I want. I'll have to start going quickly. My legs, stamina, and my willingness to be active are diminishing. I still have my handwriting and the ability to type as I'm doing now is still holding up.

Recently walking has become so difficult at certain times of each day, usually late afternoons, that I brought in my walker from the car. Oh, where is the old me that I was? I'm not happy that I can no longer do anything that requires a balance, that delicious feeling that we all take for granted. I haven't fallen so far but feel it coming on. This morning I got up as usual around 7:00 and first on my mind I asked for Dr. Kevorkian. I got a chuckle. Hee-hee. I've watched movies with more suspense than this. Now at the **end of May** I'm suffering. My legs are very weak. My dyskinesia mixed in with arthritis is so obnoxiously obvious that hiding my symptoms is not possible. With my cane in hand I meet so many good neighbors everywhere who ask if they can help. I don't mind those helpers. But, crap, I would still like to have a lady friend to be with.

Until this book is finished I am not ready for assisted living or any like facility. I'd like to feel I have a choice. Of course, as it's been going, I will have no real choice. The shudder in my footsteps is very annoying. At least I didn't get the tremor back in my left hand.

Oh where, oh where did MOM go? I was able to control the Parkinson's appearance until several months ago. I work to get my Mind-Over-Matter back though I find it more difficult this time. And to that I say, "CRAP." My bowling game hasn't suffered as I thought it would; muscle use has not diminished as I thought it would have. I bowl twice a week. Once I get my legs straight I will get back to golf.

Since I brought the walker in from the trunk, I refuse to cave to the use of it. I feel when I do I will be conceding; that the disease has won. When I can no longer get around on my own, I feel I will have lost the battle.

NOTE: In the last week of August, 2014 Robin Williams, Actor/Comedian, ended his life. The next day we found out he had Parkinson's. A few days later one of our PD members, in a wheelchair, ended his life. It's a terrible disease that we have to have the strength to endure and but not do anything extreme.

August 31, 2014. This may be the end of my tale. I have no strength in my body to get up and my urine is red. I always said no hospital unless I'm bleeding. I never considered bleeding internally. But I might be. I got in my recliner and three hours later I felt the everyday bad, never good. The bad news, I'm going to live.

There might be what seems like some duplication as you read. It's over two years since I started writing and I want some sleep. The sleeping difficulty may never go away. I've just gotten arthritis across my shoulder making it very painful in the back of my neck and it's preventing my turning over in bed without the devastating pain. I wear a foam neck brace but it becomes too hot in a short time. It's a relief to remove it but then it's back to the pain. Since September began I've had this dreadful neck pain more discomforting than PD. It's like I had been taking Viagra and all I got was a stiff neck.

If I can't return to my computer, I want you all to know I love you for reading this. Most of all I love Sheila for being my friend and working on the book with me to complete lest it come to a premature end. I can't possibly know when the end may be. Until then, you stay well and enjoy living your life. I continue to enjoy my life with the accomplishment of this book.

One exception. A new development has

raised its ugly head and, with general weakness of both legs, has caused me to fall on four different occasions recently. As we are constantly reminded, Parkinson's is a progressive disease.

Book #2

For Women

"Life is what happens~~

~~when you have other plans."

Sheila Feige

SHEILA

Ed Kluft searched extensively and finally chose me to write the book for women. I initially felt the time needed was too difficult to fit into my schedule. However, he was quite persuasive—he did all but get on his knees to plead. I accepted and became co-author.

My name is Sheila Feige. I was born in Michigan City, IN, in October of 1939. I now live in The Villages. It's a retirement community for people over the age of 55. There are support groups for every need listed in our newspaper, *The Daily Sun*. It was here where I met Ed Kluft at one of the support groups for Parkinson's and he asked me to co-author his book on this disease. At first I thought, "Oh no, I simply can't give that much time and effort." Then, after further reflection, I came to the conclusion that maybe, just maybe, I might be able to help others get through some of the scary thoughts you have with this condition.

So, here goes! My book about my 21+ years with Parkinson's Disease.

I've been a healthy individual most of my life. I had all the childhood diseases and my share of colds and flu. Things I have always done and still love to do are dancing and exercising. It is by far always more fun to do those with a partner. I remember some of the dances I did while in high school. I seemed to be able to catch on to the steps very quickly and usually ended up teaching my classmates how to do them. I feel that the dancing and exercising has helped slow down the advance of Parkinson's.

In the first year of being diagnosed with PD, all I really had was the tremor in my left leg. It was at this time that I experienced a great deal of embarrassment. Even though I knew I wasn't at fault, I still felt "funny". I did everything I could to cover up that shaking. To this day, I still have a hang up and try to mask the tremors. When I go out on the golf course and am teeing off, I will start that old shaking and I usually turn toward my golfing friends and simply say "Parkinson's, I hate it." They all understand. I have never requested any help while playing golf and I usually try to walk as much of the course as I can. I consider playing golf part of my exercise for that day. I was put on the "Grand Daddy" medication for Parkinson's treatment. It is Sinemet (25/100) 1pill every 3 hours or the generic Carbidopa/Levodopa. This drug is one of the first to have been prescribed for PD and it still is the most effective one of all.

Sinemet has helped me to manage my shaking. After being on it for a short while, I still was getting tremors, especially at night. I mentioned this to my doctor and he then added another drug, Requip (4 mg) 3 times per day which reduced the symptoms that were bothering me. I have stayed with these pills the entire time I have had PD. Every once in a while the doctor will ask me to try another medication but I always have a reaction. The reactions I seem to get are usually diarrhea or stomach aches.

Of all the symptoms one can get if they have PD, I started with only one, *tremors*. I have never experienced on/off time until just recently. I have learned over the years that with each new symptom you must try to evaluate what you can do to lessen that symptom. I started to research PD the same day that I received my third diagnosis confirming that I did indeed have Parkinson's. The internet is the perfect place to get the latest info on PD. The more you learn about the disease you have the better equipped you are to fight it. There is a lot to be said in the phrase "the power of positive thinking". There is an old children's story written around 1930, *The Little Engine That Could*. I think we all know how the story ends. The little steam engine repeats the words, "I think I can. I think I can" and is successful at last pulling the train up the steep hill. If your mind tells you to give up, you will lose the fight against PD; but if your mind truly believes you can slow the progress down, you will have won the battle. We all know that as of this date there is no cure for Parkinson's. However, there are ways to control your symptoms.

The sense of smell is one of the first to go. Since I have always had a problem with my sinuses, this did not bother me that much. I learned that my sinuses could predict the weather for me. Whenever there was going to be a large change in the temperature or that rain, snow, heat, etc. was on its way, I would get a very severe sinus headache. Now that PD has caused the loss of smell, the sinus headaches have disappeared.

My speech started to get lower and softer. At first I thought I sounded sexy and that was great! However, when people started to say "What?" whenever I spoke to them, I realized that I had to do something. By researching in depth on the internet, I found answers as to what I should do to strengthen my voice. I was able to improve the clarity and volume. At this time there is just one person who has a devil of a time hearing me, my husband, Gary. He wears hearing aids and his hearing is getting worse. I try to remember to turn towards him when I talk to him. Some of my friends have kidded me that it's probably selective hearing on Gary's part.

Balance problems have not bothered me so far. The only thing I have experienced on a daily basis is the problem of putting on my panties and any article of clothing that has legs (such as jeans). The first time I nearly went on my rear end was when I was putting on a pair of pants. I started with my right leg. No problem! Then I put my left leg in. I thought I had it right but when I started to walk, I realized I had put my left leg in the same opening that my right leg was in. Yikes! I did a fancy two step and was successful at not falling down. It's funny now but wasn't when it was happening. Now I am very careful to get both openings open before I start to get into them. Every once in a while I seem to stagger but it's not the same as losing your balance.

It's becoming a little difficult to put makeup on when I am in a shaking mode. Eye makeup is the worst! The eye liner always goes on crooked and I have to repair the line. The mascara is another problem. I've put the brush in my eye countless times and it's not fun! I don't usually apply a lot of makeup so it's not too bad. When I put my makeup on, I use the same time to make faces at myself in the mirror. This helps eliminate the frozen face look of the "Parkinson mask". I find that smiling is the best one of all.

My posture is beginning to get stiff looking and I try to loosen it up with my hand held weights when I exercise. I believe the PD terminology is rigidity.

I have always had a problem with constipation and diarrhea. It isn't something new to me. Diet and lots of liquids (especially water) really help. This symptom works on both genders. Miralax is my choice when I am constipated. I was told by my PCP that you can take it every day without worrying about its becoming habit forming. Still you can swing from constipation to diarrhea when you take a laxative. So, it's damned if you do and damned if you don't.

Women are infamous for trying to lose weight and to get that "Barbie Doll" look. Well, guess what? If you are one of the unlucky ones that contract Parkinson's, you just might wind up with abdominal distention or bloating. In plain English, a big belly! If you should get the stooped look in your shoulders in addition to the big belly, you will have what we call the "S" shape. This is not pretty. Unfortunately it is sometimes unavoidable because of good old PD. The loss of weight is a common occurrence in PD and it usually levels off after having the disease for some time. The norm for people with PD is to stay thin rather than be a heavyweight. This does not help wrinkles or saggy skin.

1994—Whoa! I just realized that I am getting ahead of myself in this story; so I will start at the point when it all began. 1994 was the year a dream came true and a nightmare started.

I always had a wish for a Corvette and my husband said "You only go around once. Why don't you make yourself happy and buy one?" So the top item on my "bucket list" became a reality for me. It was a beautiful red car. Very powerful and very fast. After getting my car, I began to notice that I was starting to shake. I thought that maybe it was my new car making me nervous. A blonde in a red Corvette brought out all the macho men to challenge me to see if they could beat me off the line.

For 25 years I had been employed by the same company, Marvin L. Walker & Assoc. Inc., as the Director of Human Resources. The job was hectic at times but I am an individual who loves a challenge. In plain English, I loved my job. One morning while I was standing at the copier, one of my coworkers said to me "Sheila, do you know that your left leg always shakes when you are standing still?" I told her I was still getting used to my car and that I felt it was probably nerves. I felt very self-conscious knowing that people were noticing that damn tremor. When I got back to my desk, I picked up the phone to schedule a visit with my PCP. It was time for my annual check-up anyway. During my appointment, they performed all the usual procedures—blood pressure, urinalysis, blood drawn for several different tests, etc.

They asked if there was anything that I wanted to discuss with the doctor so I told them about the tremor. When the doctor addressed my question, he said he had noticed the shaking but that it was very minor and probably just nerves. I told him about my guess that my new car was the reason for making me nervous. He then told me that if I was that uneasy driving a sports car, maybe I should trade it in for an "old lady car." Did I mention that he could be a real cut-up? So I told him where he could put that idea. At this point in time no diagnosis for Parkinson's had been made.

Sometime after that appointment, our company changed their insurance provider and my PCP wasn't on the new plan. I picked out a new one and made an appointment right away so I could meet him to see if I liked him. Although I did not say anything about the tremor, he had noticed and asked me about it. He said to me, "I would like you to see a neurologist and talk to him about the tremor." I asked him if there was anything I should be concerned about. He said he just wanted to be thorough.

The next week I saw a neurologist. After our initial conversation, he gave me some strange tests

- walking up and down the hallway,
- pushing me forward and backward,
- opening and closing my fingers as quickly as I could,
- slapping my thigh, etc.

Later, I found out from other Parkinsonians that they had been tested in the same way.

After completion of these tests, the neurologist told me there was a possibility of Parkinson's disease. Before he would give me a positive diagnosis, he wanted to line up an MRI with contrast of my brain. Since I had no earthly idea of what Parkinson's disease was, he had just scared the shit out of me. MRI??? Brain???? Now I really was nervous. I asked him to explain Parkinson's. He said it was a neurological disorder and gave me the explanation in medical terms. Since I was still in the dark (not understanding the medical terms), he suggested I go home and search the internet to get a more thorough explanation. He told me not to research too deeply until they ruled out other possibilities after the MRI was done.

The day of the MRI arrived. It wasn't at all bad. The technician asked me if it were possible for me to stop shaking and I answered him, "Yes, but you'll have to kill me to get the shaking to stop." If you've never had an MRI, it can be scary. Fortunately, I can tolerate small spaces and very loud noises. If you get the MRI with contrast, you go through the procedure in the tube twice. The first time before and the second time after the radioactive contrast agent is injected. After making sure that all metal objects (jewelry, watches, belts, change, etc.) have been removed from your body, they lay you on a very narrow padded table. This is to make your back comfortable. After they get you situated by stabilizing your head so that it doesn't move during the procedure and by propping up your knees with a pillow, you are rolled into a very narrow opening in a gigantic tube. Some medical facilities offer head phones with music and some even have a mirror that you can look into and see the technicians monitoring you. However, if you get scared by confined spaces, you may have a problem getting the test done. It's best to tell the technicians before the test begins so they are prepared to make changes. They keep you informed during the whole test on what is happening, what you will experience, how long it will take, etc. Once you are in the tube, they start the MRI. The noise is almost indescribable. It sounds as if someone has a wrench and is pounding it on the outside of the tube. First a slow tap that gradually goes up to an extremely loud and very rapid pace. They give you instructions before the test begins that include not talking, breathing loudly and trying not to swallow. That's the funny one. "Don't swallow?" Well, you know that when you are told not to swallow, it makes it next to impossible not to get a bunch of saliva building up in your mouth. You have to swallow because you know you will drown in your own spit if you don't. So, I thought it through and swallowed in slow motion. Hey, good for me, it worked!

The next day my husband and I went to get the results of the MRI. The doctor told us that the test did not show anything abnormal and with that information he confirmed his diagnosis that I had Parkinson's. He then told us he had one other test he wanted to do. He was going to give me a pill called Sinemet. He wanted me to take the pill to see if it would alleviate the shaking. If it did, we could rest assured that the diagnosis was correct. Then, we would discuss which medication to start me on.

I could not believe what I was hearing. Why would I have contracted Parkinson's? No one in my family had ever had it and I was sure I didn't do anything to start it. I kept thinking I had been misdiagnosed. I was in a state of denial. I voiced all this to my husband. He responded, "What would you like to do about it?" I answered, "See another doctor!" I then made an appointment with the second neurologist who also came with good qualifications. I waited almost two weeks before seeing the new doctor. I spent these two weeks on the internet doing some serious research. The time spent in his office almost exactly mirrored my first appointment. The tests were the same. I was very open with this doctor. I let him know I was there to get a second opinion. After about an hour, he said he agreed with the first doctor and that the diagnosis was correct. I still did not believe it was true. Did I tell you that I am a doubting Thomas and always want proof of everything before I believe it? These doctors were not giving me the proof I needed to believe that I, Sheila Feige, could have contracted PD.

After leaving the doctor's office, I voiced my concern to Gary. He asked me what the next step should be. I was at a loss. I spent the day in tears and frustration. Why me???? I had not told anyone else about the PD as I was going to buckle down and do further research online before I opened up to anyone.

Gary was my strength at this time. He ran

our dry cleaning business in Gainesville, GA, where our clientele were mostly professional people: bankers, dentists, doctors, accountants, etc. Gary came home that night and said he had talked to several customers and had asked them if they knew of a doctor who was a leader in Parkinson's. Several people mentioned a neurologist, Dr. Ray Watts, who worked at Emory University in Atlanta. This doctor was supposed to be the #1 neurologist for Parkinson's. He had great credentials. This is when I told Gary to make the appointment for me to see this doctor and if he agreed with the first two, I would cease to doubt that I had Parkinson's.

When I met the new doctor, I liked him immediately. He was the leading neurologist at Emory. His wife worked with him in the Neurological Department. He gave me the same round of tests that the other two doctors had given me. I decided that there is no precise test to prove that one has PD. I retained Dr. Watts for a good many years until he accepted an offer from the University of Alabama—Birmingham where he was to run the entire Movement Disorder, Neurological Department. He has written several books, articles and has made several appearances on TV. This man took a lot of time with me and in the end he agreed with the other two doctors that I did indeed have PD. Depression set in almost as soon as those words came out of his mouth. He asked me what medications I had tried so far. I told him that I had tried several, including one that was the cause of my not being able to urinate.

That was a day from hell. My bladder was so full I felt it was going to burst. I rushed to see a urologist and I specifically asked him if this symptom could be caused by the new medication I had just started for my PD. He looked up the medication and told me no it wouldn't cause that symptom. Being the doubting Thomas that I am, I stopped the medication on my own and the problem was solved. Later that day I researched this drug and the inability to urinate was one of the side effects listed. So much for doctors always giving their patients the right answers. This is one thing I would caution anyone starting a new medication. Do read the side effects of the medicine. Had I been smart enough to do this first, I would have saved myself a lot of stress, a trip to a urologist and the money it cost to see him.

Dr. Watts never pulled any punches. He was always honest with his answers to my questions. He told me I should look up support groups. I never followed that suggestion because I knew that my job would not allow me to take the time off. In my research on this disease, I found that there are quite a few different types and symptoms of PD. Mine seemed to be just the <u>essential tremors and dyskinesia</u>, which is an involuntary body motion from side to side. I thanked God and still do for giving me the PD that is advancing slowly. I have been told by many people that they cannot tell that I have PD. I'm one of the lucky ones whose symptoms do not show so far.

The next day at work I called a meeting with my supervisors and told them everything that had been going on and that I had PD. They both expressed that they had not noticed any symptoms of PD and as long as I could perform my duties, they had no problem with it at all. I continued this job until I reached the age of 70. I hated it when my tremors would pick up when I had to be involved in a meeting. There were days when I just couldn't control the shaking. I always felt as if everyone in the room was focusing on me. Most of the time I felt very obvious. I became self-conscious. I learned the trick of sitting on my hands. This seemed to help in slowing down the shaking, which made me feel much better.

Throughout the years since diagnosis, Gary has decided not to do anything for me that he knows I am able to do. I'm a firm believer that if the Parkinson's patient accepts all help, whether they need it or not, they will accelerate the development Parkinson's. Not only that, but I feel they will be better off mentally knowing that they are still a functioning human being.

Gary and I have had only one area where we have disagreed. He became a complete pest about reminding me to take my medicine on time. I would set the alarm on my cell phone and it would remind me that it was time. I always heard it but if I were in the middle of a project, I would delay taking my medicine until I was finished.

In the meantime, Gary would also hear it and yell to me, "Have you taken your medicine?" I'd yell back, "Not yet." He then would get up and march in to me and tell me, "Sheila, go take your medicine now. It should be priority." That scenario got to be old very fast. Finally, I asked him to stop being my alarm. I let

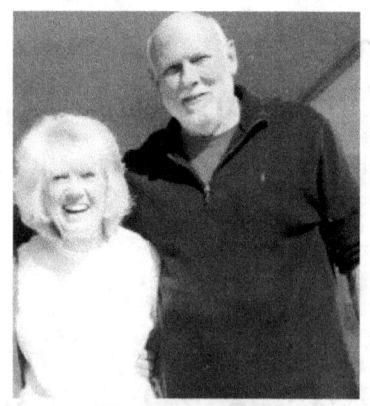

Sheila and Gary

him know that I was responsible for taking my medicine on time. I told him that maybe someday I would really need his help and I would appreciate it then. He finally agreed. To this day, I am responsible for my meds. Gary is my care giver but because I am not in great need, he really has not had that much to do.

Gary has always been the type of person who is willing to share the chores around the house and I've always been thankful for that.

My appointments with my doctor occurred on average every six months. My medicine never changed and it worked well for me. I took Sinemet (Carbidopa/Levodopa 25/100) four times per day and Requip (Ropinirole 4 mg) three times per day. I remember the doctor telling me that if I found a drug or a combination of drugs that worked well for me, not to change them. Changing to a different drug might work against me and cause a change in the slow movement of my PD.

When my doctor left for his new position in Birmingham, he sent all my records to another neurologist at Emory whom he had recommended. I really liked this doctor. She was on the ball. She was still in her studies while having a full practice at Emory University. She asked me if I would take part in one of her clinical trials on the effect of Vitamin B-12 on Parkinson's symptoms. She explained that I would be in the hospital overnight and taken off all meds until the next afternoon. This was for testing purposes. I agreed knowing that it was strictly for the knowledge they would get through testing. The first tests started immediately when I entered the hospital at around 2PM. All my meds were taken away. The doctor came in again around 6PM and told me that she would be in the next morning around 9AM to do the second round of tests. She cautioned me not to take any PD medication. My tremors started to pick up in the evening. If you've ever been in a hospital overnight, you know it is almost impossible to sleep. Even with the door closed to your room from the hallway, there is still light and noise entering the room. You can even hear conversations between nurses, aides, and hospital personnel. At around 3AM a young hospital aide came into my room and said it was time for me to take my PD meds. I then explained to him why I was there and the one thing that I was told not to do was to take any PD meds. I told him it would completely destroy the test. He told me that it was on my chart to give me the meds. I told him, "No way! I'm following the doctor's orders that she has given me." He said he would make a note on my chart that I had refused the meds. The next morning the doctor arrived promptly at 9AM. I told her about the aide coming in during the night and my conversation with him. She was so thankful that I had refused the meds and made a note to talk to the aide's supervisor. I told her that it was a good thing that I couldn't sleep. If I had been sound asleep when he came in, I might have been too groggy to know what was going on and taken the medicine. The tests went as planned and lasted about one to two hours. At around noon I was discharged with either a Vitamin B-12 placebo or the real thing. I was not told which one I had been given. One month later I was given a list of questions to fill out. I never learned the outcome of that study.

I remember one 8AM appointment with the doctor. Gary and I always tried to get the first appointment in the morning so that I could go to work without breaking up the day. That morning we were the first ones in the outer waiting room which serviced about six different doctors. We had just sat down when another couple came in to see my doctor with an 8:15AM appointment. The lady was in a wheelchair and her husband was pushing her. She was in advanced stages of PD. We were both called in to go to our exam rooms at the same time. While we were waiting to see the doctor, we could hear the doctor's PA talking to the couple who had come in after us. I told my husband that I thought we would have been first since I had the earlier appointment. Within five minutes, the doctor's PA came into our room and said "Sheila Feige?" I said "Yes." She started laughing and went on to tell us that the person who puts the patients in the exam rooms to see the doctor had gotten us mixed up with the couple that had the 8:15 appointment. She had made a mistake and put the other patient in the room I was supposed to be in and had put me in the other patient's room. The PA walked into the room with my file expecting to see me with notes stating how wonderful I was doing and instead, was looking at the lady in the wheelchair. She said to Gary and me, "My God, I wondered what could have happened to cause that much deterioration in such a short time. When I called out your name the husband told me that Sheila was not his wife's name." It was a good way to start the day. We laugh every time we think of that mix-up.

After seeing this doctor for about 1½ years, she let us know that she was quitting her practice and devoting her time to finishing her schooling. I was beginning to think that I was not going to have any luck in keeping a good doctor. Every time I knew I had an excellent one, they left. So, it was back to the search mode for a new doctor. Gary and I talked it over and decided to look for one in our area. Gainesville is a regional medical hub for Northeast Georgia. The medical facilities are superb and it draws excellent physicians and technicians. After talking to quite a few of our dry cleaning customers, I decided on Dr. M. B., who is the spitting image of Dr. McDreamy (Patrick Dempsey) on Grey's Anatomy. Not that his looks had anything to do with my choice. It did make my appointments a lot easier to take. Just think, ladies, looking into the eyes of Dr. McDreamy just inches from your face. His qualifications and mannerisms were of the highest professional standards. So, once again, I had chosen a good one! He remained my doctor for the duration of the time we lived in Georgia. Then came the move to The Villages in Florida.

In my original researching I had discovered that most of the articles written on PD had a common thread on how to slow down the progress of the disease: exercise with music. This was right up my alley. I have been an exercise nut my entire life. I love music; so putting the two together made sense. Every day I would make it my goal to get at least a half hour of exercise in. I put together a series of exercises which would target those areas of my body that had a tendency to gain weight. These areas vary for women but in my case, it was my tummy and hips. I had always wanted to discover a way to push the fat up from my stomach to my breasts but it never happened. I was small boned and the most I ever weighed was 130 lbs. That was in my first pregnancy in 1962. I could have kept that weight down but I was "eating for two". Remember that stupid statement? I consumed a lot of doughnuts during my first pregnancy. I remember the clothes I took with me to the hospital to wear on the trip home with my brand new son, Scott. I had decided on a pair of jeans and a sweat shirt. But when it was time to get dressed to take the trip home, I started to put on the pair of jeans and guess what! They didn't fit!! All those doughnuts stared at me through a very fat stomach. I had a span of about three inches in front that was open and I couldn't get those jeans to close. So, I had to send Ron home to get a pair of sweat pants. I started to cry and didn't stop for almost an hour. Depression set in. So did my determination to lose those extra pounds and the exercising started. My second son, Mark, was born 3½ years later. And I went home that time with less weight on my body than I had before I got pregnant. I had learned my lesson.

They say that stress is one of the worst things for your health. I have put together a partial list of very stressful periods that I experienced in my lifetime.

1) In my early 30s I had pain and internal swelling resulting from a hole that had developed in my rectum wall. In those days they did not have laser surgery so the surgery to repair the hole was done on the operating table. The surgeon had to cut my sphincter muscle to be able to reach the hole. I have lived the rest of my life with a break in that all important muscle. Remember that muscle controls your ability to hold the gas that we all pass in any day. It has caused me a great deal of embarrassment and how do I explain it???

2) My first husband, Ron, developed Hodgkin's disease (cancer of the lymphatic system) while he was in his 30s. We took him for daily treatments and radiation at the Billings Hospital in Chicago, IL, which was about a 70 mile drive from Michigan

City, IN. We were very fortunate that the treatments were successful in putting the Hodgkin's into remission.

3) My father passed away at the age of 59 from cancer of the lungs. He had smoked his whole life. This created another problem – my mother had never learned to drive. I taught her to drive at the age of 58.

4) Ron passed away in 1982 at the age of 42 from a blood clot lodged in the artery to his heart. His arteries had narrowed due to the radiation given to him for his Hodgkin's disease and the clot couldn't pass. He was on the tennis court playing tennis with our youngest son, Mark, when he died. Mark did not play tennis for a couple of years after that.

5) I married a man whom I met in my job with Designhouse Intl. I thought all marriages ended in a happy state. I found out different. He cheated on me from the start. That marriage lasted only a year. I filed for divorce and it was shortly after that that I met and married Gary Cook.

6) Our house on Lake Lanier in Gainesville, GA, caught on fire and burned on Christmas Eve, 2009. It took about six months to rebuild it.

7) My mother suffered a mild stroke and developed heart disease. She died at the age of 85.

8) In the late 90s my husband, Gary developed a perforation in his lower intestines and had to have emergency surgery. The surgery removed a section of his colon and because of the infection he had to have a colostomy put in until it cleared up. The doctor told Gary that it would be about six months before they could reconnect his intestines. Five months later Gary was back to normal. He will tell you that it was the longest five months in his life. If we had not gotten Gary to the hospital, the doctors told us, he would have died from the infection.

9) Six months after Gary's first surgery, he had to have a second surgery to repair a hernia which had developed due to the

first surgery.

10)   In 2006 Gary was diagnosed with Prostate Cancer. We were given several options to choose from and finally decided to have the prostate removed. It has been successful in that all of his follow-up tests since then have showed no signs of the cancer.

11)   In 2010 Holly, our pet cat, had to be put down because she had lost the use of her rear legs. She was eighteen and was a beautiful brown tabby. She had developed a disease of the heart muscle called "Hypertrophic cardiomyopathy". This disease causes blood clots to form within the chambers of the heart. If one breaks free, it circulates rapidly and lodges in an artery supplying blood to the rear legs. Sudden paralysis is the consequences. I still am upset by her death but she had a good life with us.

There are many other situations that have caused stress in my life but the above are the ones that stand out in my mind. I have decided to follow the advice in the Serenity Prayer. It says:

> God, grant me the serenity to accept the things I cannot change, the courage to change the things I can, and the wisdom to know the difference.

And also, the title of my portion of this book, "Life is what happens when you have other plans". This saying was one that Ron used a lot. I met Ron while going to High School. We lived in Michigan City, IN, which is at the tip of Lake Michigan. We were fifteen years of age when we met. It was love at first sight. It was actually the second time we had met. In the old days when women delivered their babies, they stayed for ten days in the hospital. I was born on October 16 and Ron was born on October 25 in the same hospital. My mother knew Ron's mother and they ran into each other on the day of Ron's birth. My mother was taking me home the next day. Ron and I were in the same room in the hospital for one day.

We met in the summer of 1955 on the beautiful beach of Lake Michigan, graduated in 1957, and married in October of 1959. Scott (our first son) was born in October of 1962 and Mark (our second son) was born in December of 1965. Ron died in May of 1982 and I thank God for the wonderful years we had together. We did not smoke, we did not drink, and both of us exercised. So, the questions remain: "Why did he get Hodgkin's and why did I get Parkinson's?"

After Ron's death in 1982, I went to work immediately. After a few years and one divorce, I filed for a mortgage on a townhouse in Duluth, GA. That's how I met Gary Cook, a mortgage originator and real estate broker. It was during the application for my mortgage that Gary and I found we had several things in common. The biggest was our love for sailing. Gary was the Racing Commodore for the Lanier Sailing Club. During the application for my mortgage, he asked me if I had ever entered my boat in a night race. I had never raced my boat at any time. He then asked me if I would crew for him on his boat on the next night race. I then asked him the all-important question, "Are you married?" He told me "No I'm divorced." So I agreed to be part of his crew. Gary and I raced our boat, Mon Cherie (My Darling) many times, brought home quite a few trophies, spent quite a few weekends on the boat and got married three months later.

2009: Gary and I had been talking about retirement and where to retire. Our home in Gainesville, GA, was right on Lake Lanier. It was just a summer cottage that the previous owners had used when they wanted outings on the lake. Gary at that time was a real estate broker and had taken me out to look at this "cottage" which was for sale. We arrived just as the sun was beginning to set. I fell in love with it immediately.

I've already mentioned that our lake house burned down on Christmas Eve. I did not mention that we had just completed a seven-month renovation. That night we had our first fire in our wood burning fireplace. Around midnight, Gary said, "Get up, Sheila, we've got a fire". I opened my eyes to a room full of smoke. We threw on sweat suits, grabbed a few things, and got out of the house. It was very cold that morning and the water from the firemen's hoses was freezing on the front driveway as it ran down to the street.

So, we started all over again. After five months of reconstruction, we moved back into our home. Throughout our years there, we continuously improved the house (and added to the mortgage). The years started to go by and my Parkinson's had been diagnosed. Through those passing of years, it was beginning to take its toll. On the busy commute to and from work, I started to get terribly sleepy while driving. The reason? The Ropinirole! It was beginning to have a narcoleptic effect on me. I started to fall asleep with no forewarning at all. I could be wide awake one minute and sound asleep the next. Gary and I discussed this and he started to drive me back and forth to work every day. It was at this time that we realized that it was time to think about retirement. We really wanted to enjoy some quality years before it became too late. We started to go on short three day trips to visit various retirement communities. After about six months we decided that we really wanted to move to Florida.

The biggest draw was the warm weather all year round. We put our dry cleaning business up for sale and found a buyer. In November of 2009 we put our house up for sale. We asked my cousin and her husband, Bev & Keith Nichols, about retirement communities, told us they had purchased a home in The Villages in Florida and lived there for six months of every year. They said it was simply wonderful with all types of activities. We immediately lined up a trip to see and gather information on The Villages. We were very impressed. I fell in love with one Designer Home plan, "The Lantana". We placed a down payment on a lot in the Village of Bonita. It was fun going through the decisions of what to put in the house as our home would be built according to the choices we made.

Up to this time my Parkinson's did not bother me much. The only time it seemed to raise its ugly head was when I would get stressed. And it would manifest itself in the form of shaking. It was at this time that I noticed my voice was beginning to sound softer or lower. I thought it was a sexy sound but when people began to say "What?" or "Excuse me but I didn't hear you", I knew I had to start working on it or I would lose it.

In September, 2010, we moved into our new home. Our neighbors were simply wonderful. They all came at different times to introduce themselves. There were 18 homes on Columbia Way and all were permanent year-round residents. No snow birds!

One of the first things I got out of the way was to tell each one of my neighbors that I have Parkinson's. It didn't seem to bother them at all. My regiment of exercise stopped at this time due to the fact that I was getting a work out just getting the house decorated and in order. At the end of each day, Gary and I were exhausted. The movers had done a great job in placing the boxes in the correct rooms but the enormous task of placing all the packed items in their proper places was at times overwhelming. We also went shopping for new furniture for certain rooms but that job was fun.

It was at this time that the job of picking out new doctors and dentists began. We relied heavily on word of mouth. Our next door neighbors, A.J. & Diane Monacelli, gave us the name of the dentist that they were using. We took it without hesitation since A.J.'s previous profession had been dentist. No one had the name of a neurologist so Gary and I went to the yellow pages and the internet. We chose a neurologist who seemed to have a large patient following. I liked him immediately. Through the initial conversation with him, we found out that he had studied under Dr. Ray Watts, my doctor at Emory University in Atlanta. After examining me and running me through those goofy tests, he made the observation that he could not tell that I had Parkinson's from my actions. He questioned as to whether I really had Parkinson's. He then gave me orders to try an experiment and stop all medications to see what my reactions would be. I was willing to give it a try.

I tried and it failed!!! I was shaking so hard when I went back to see him that he commented if Dr. Ray Watts had diagnosed me with Parkinson's, he would not question it. He thinks the world of Dr. Watts. After that visit, I always have seen his PA who is very knowledgeable. During the time that I have been in The Villages, the PA has put me on different medications to see if I would be better. They never work. Every time I've tried a new medicine, I remember Dr. Ray Watt's words to me, "If you find a drug or a combination of drugs that works, DO NOT CHANGE. Sometimes that experiment can work against you." He'd gone on to explain that some medicines for some people can do damage and the Parkinson's accelerates.

Since my move to Florida, I have had a swallow test as one of the symptoms of Parkinson's is the inability to swallow. The results of the swallow test were that my esophagus narrows and I could get food stuck there if I'm not careful. Quite frequently when I am drinking a beverage, it goes down into my wind pipe and I wind up coughing my head off trying to clear the fluid. Now that's scary. I have nightmares about choking to death. The doctors suggest taking smaller bite-sized pieces of food and chewing the food very well.

My neurologist suggested that I take the tests from the Memory Doctor to check my memory. I went in 2013 and again in 2014. I was very pleased when the results came back stating that my memory had improved from 2013 to 2014. My understanding is that with Parkinson's you develop memory loss. I am developing this memory loss in things like, "Where did I put my medicine for the day?" And I wind up spending a lot of time looking for things I have misplaced. I wonder if it's just old age or the Parkinson's. I do crazy things that I don't remember doing. I have the misfortune of being one of the people who fall asleep without any warning. This is one of the side effects of Requip or Ropinirole.

However, I have stopped driving a car due to the effect of Requip. It finally came to a crisis one Sunday in February. I attended the afternoon Fight Club. I had driven myself to the meeting because Gary was working as an Ambassador for one of the men he works with on the Arnold Palmer golf courses. After the meeting ended, I started to drive myself home. We have a 2008 Cadillac CTS and it just about drives itself. The snow birds were still in the Villages which made traffic heavier. I was in the habit of setting the Cruise Control on Buena Vista at 39mph. The speed limit is 35mph. I was fully awake when I started to drive home but I had taken my Ropinirole and it kicked in. Buena Vista is a four lane street with a median of grass, trees, flowers, etc. I had just about reached The Village of Bridgeport—Lake Sumter when I dropped into a deep sleep like a narcoleptic. The next thing I was aware of was the car coming down on all four wheels. I remember my nose hitting the steering wheel and when my eyes opened, I was facing oncoming traffic. I remember thinking "What the hell are all these cars doing on my side of the road?" In the blink of an eye, I knew I was on their side of the road. The car stopped on its own, well, with the help of my foot on the brake. I suddenly realized I had fallen asleep; but with the grace of God, I had not hit anyone or anything and had not injured myself.

A lady who lived in the neighborhood had been in her golf cart on the golf cart path. She came running over and put me through several small tests to make sure I was all right. She told me she had seen the whole thing and that my car had actually gone air borne over the center median. The oncoming traffic had all come to a stop and could not move until I moved my car which meant doing a U-turn. That was extremely difficult because when the car had come down on the opposite side, I blew all four tires out and flattened all four wheels. But I took it slowly and with some maneuvering back and forth, I turned the car around and pulled into the Village of Bridgeport. I called Gary and he was there with me within a half hour. Brenda stayed with me until he arrived. I want to thank Brenda once again as she was very concerned about me and I am so grateful she stayed until Gary arrived. We called AAA and since there were no injuries or any damage (with the exception of my car) we did not involve the police. My car did not touch the median at all and I can't tell you how the devil it cleared the median but it did. This is one time when I am sure God put an angel in the car with me because I know I had help to avoid a catastrophe. Needless to say I made the decision to give up driving the car and I am sticking to it. All my neighbors have nicknamed me "Crash Feige". I won't even tell you how much that repair on the Cadillac cost me but it was a bunch!

When I began seeing my neurologist, he and his PA suggested that since I was doing so well with PD, I should check into one of the support groups for Parkinson's. I had never been interested in support groups because, quite frankly, I didn't really need one yet. I seemed to be one of the lucky (????) people with Parkinson's that has a slow moving progression. Up to that time I had not done any research into the support groups but the PA continued to remind me about them. I finally decided to give it a try when she said to me "Sheila, with your outgoing personality and the fact that you seem to have a handle on the PD, I feel you could be a big help to the people that attend the support groups. So, please consider joining, as a gift from you." That's all it took. I told her I would look into it right away. *The Daily Sun* has a weekly insert that lists all the clubs and support groups available to all residents of The Villages. I found two support groups that held meetings in the Villages.

I attended the meeting for the "Parkinson's' Thursday Exercise/Support Group". It has a very warm group of about 30+ people and their very intelligent leaders. I felt very comfortable there. Meetings feature several different types of exercises: both standing and sitting to music, working with stretch bands, yoga, speech therapy, and recreational fun things to do. In addition they play memory games which I love. The tempo of the music varies from a slow to medium beat. The individuals joining this group will tell you in a heartbeat if the music is beyond their reach. This is great for those with PD since so many are in wheel chairs and the meetings are made for them. They do their homework on the different aspects of Parkinson's and always seem to be able to bring in experts who speak to the group. Their pattern is to have a couple who attend on a regular basis plan the activities for the group for a month at a time. Then, the next couple takes over. The couple is always a Parkinsonian and his/her care giver. This is what makes this group special. It is run by a member of the group with one very lovely lady who oversees the business side of the group. She is responsible for sending out all emails with activities and news concerning Parkinson's as well as letting everyone know what the next month's agenda will be. Her emails are professional and very informative. She does not put personal information in them with items that have nothing to do with Parkinson's. With the overflow of email junk that we are sent, it's a joy to have someone stay on track.

The week after I joined the Thursday group, I went to a second support group. Unlike the first group with just one meeting per week, this one meets on Sundays and Wednesdays for the Parkinsonians and their care givers. They also meet on Monday mornings but that meeting is strictly for men. This group has a much larger following of people. Their exercise portion of the meeting is half hour of very upbeat music. The tempo and beat can be extremely fast but the group is told to go at their own pace. The other 1½ hours are usually the same for every meeting. A Parkinson's subject is brought up for discussion. The problem with that is that the answers get boring after you go through the entire room. The amount of people he has attending is almost too much for the room when they do their exercise portion.

The main leader of the group called me after my first attendance with his group and asked me if I would consider helping in the exercise portion as an example to the group of someone who had lived with PD for 18+ years. So, I began to attend the second group on a regular basis. I attended this group well over 1 ½ years before I decided to go back to the first group. The reason for the change was a personal conflict with the social director. I still retain the friendships I developed while at this second group and run into them every once in a while. They let me know that they miss me and miss my leading part of the exercise portion of the meeting. It's great to know that I did help and this makes me feel happy. In fact, several of the people with PD and their care givers are now steady friends with my husband and me. We get together about once every two weeks. Bear in mind that you can attend both meetings if you wish.

I am now involved with the Thursday group and am bringing in some new music with a variety of tempos. In addition to the Parkinson's Thursday Exercise/Support Group meeting at the Chatham Recreation Center, I attend a new group, "Women only care givers". It meets every Monday morning at the

Mulberry Recreation Center. It is run by Linda Wilkerson and Karen Eicher. Both women's husbands have Parkinson's. Women with Parkinson's are also invited to come. It is a great way for women to socialize and air their thoughts. Since I don't drive, Linda makes the trip to pick me up, which makes her an angel in my eyes. Thank you, Linda!

It is now May of 2015. I am beginning to have tremors earlier each day than in the past. The neurologist I have been seeing will tell you to do your own experimenting with your meds. So with that in mind, I am now taking one pill of Carbidopa/Levodopa 25/100 every two and a half hours. I have also cut my dosage of 4 mg. of Ropinirole to 2 mg. and take it with every dose of Carbidopa/Levodopa. I am forced to use my cell phone as an alarm to tell me it is time to take my medicine. Two and a half hours is a very short time between doses and I seem to be taking medicine all the time. I am now suffering from the following:

a) Drooling. I can still control it somewhat just by chewing gum. Of course, I wake up with wet spots on my pillow.

b) Constipation and diarrhea. It's like watching a tennis match—back and forth, back and forth, etc.

c) Hallucinations. Mine are usually strings that turn into bugs that are moving.

d) Sleep disturbances. This is the result of nightmares (some are really scary) and getting up to use the bathroom.

e) Dyskinesia. The amount has picked up. I sway and don't realize I'm doing it. I hate that.

f) Tremors. Sometimes I cannot control or slow down the tremors. At times it will start even though I have not reached the end of my two and a half hours.

It was after these symptoms were getting closer in time and quantity, I knew I could not get my present doctor to do much more for me. I felt as if he didn't really care; so I decided to try to find an exceptionally good doctor. I started asking different people whom they saw and what their feelings were concerning their doctor. One name came up over and over again—Dr. Annette Nieves. People love this doctor.

At this time I had the good fortune to attend a meeting held by one of the support groups and for which Dr. Nieves was the speaker. I was on the phone the very next day to schedule an appointment with her. However, she has so many patients that new patients will wait almost three months. I did not care. I was willing to wait. I asked them to put me on the call list if there was a cancellation. I was lucky! They called the very next week.

I have seen Dr. Nieves three times and this last time she gave me the following advice and instructions:

a) Change in medication and dosage.

b) New medication—Rytary Extended-Release Capsules (23.75/95). I take three capsules first thing in the morning, around 7 or 7:30. I take another two capsules when the tremors start. (Today I took two capsules at 3:15PM.) Right before I go to bed I am to take one tablet of Carbidopa/Levodopa ER (50/200). I do not take any Ropinirole during the day but I do take one tablet of Ropinirole ER 8 mg. This tablet lasts twenty-four hours.

c) Drink more water. I am really trying on this one since I don't like water. I've been the #1 fan of Diet Coke forever. This change should help with the constipation.

d) I also started taking Melatonin to help me get back to sleep after bathroom trips.

e) The change in Ropinirole is helping me stay awake during the day. The reduction in Ropinirole should stop the hallucinations.

f) Monitor my intake of protein on the days I have tremors. Be sure to use more salt and drink water. My blood pressure, taken twice at my last visit, was 94/62 and 100/80. It is usually on the low side, sometimes to the point where I think I may pass out.

This brings us up to the present date, August 2015, am I am still leading the group exercise. My with about a half hour of music, dancing and portion of the exercises is in the cardiovascular area. We also have a fellow

Parkinson leading a period with the stretching bands and another leading with yoga for balance. Our Thursday group has grown in size in size (which is nice) but we will strive not to let go of the closeness members develop with everyone there.

My words to all women who have been diagnosed with Parkinson's are that there is support in these groups and the knowledge that can be gained about your disease is there for the asking. I for one will take the time to talk to anyone who needs help and understanding. Do not be afraid and never give up hope. Believe in the Power of Positive Thinking. It does work.

Above all, remember "Life is what happens when you have other plans."

Bonus Section: Ann Klonicke

A Special Introduction from Sheila Feige:

<u>HOW FORTUNATE WE ARE TO HAVE THIS GRACIOUS WOMAN'S STORY!</u> There are many women I have had the great fortune to meet who have contracted Parkinson's disease. I wanted to incorporate just one woman's story in my book for you to read and get to know. Without a doubt Ann Klonicke won that award. She doesn't wallow in self-pity but picks herself up after every incident and goes on with her life. She shows the true meaning of "Life is what happens when you have other plans."

I thank you, Ann, for being so gracious to take the time and effort to tell us the story of your life with the dreaded Parkinson's disease. While reading Ann's story, the words "Someone always has it worse than you" came to my mind. This fits Ann so well. She is a unique woman who has the tenacity to continue on despite the obstacles she has encountered.

I met Ann at the Parkinson's' Thursday Exercise/Support Group and found her to be a truly lovely lady with a beautiful smile. She is an outstanding example of the kind of person we with PD should strive to follow. I also want to thank Steve, Ann's husband of over fifty years for the love and commitment he has given Ann during her PD years. You are a special person. Both of you know the true meaning of the words "in sickness and in health".

I am proud to be able to consider Ann my friend. Please read and enjoy her story.

~~Sheila Feige

ANN'S STORY
August 2014

My story began on a sunny Sunday in August way back in 1939. I was the second child that Edward and Ruth Donnelly gave birth to. I was welcomed into the family that at that time had one other child, my sister Jane, who is almost four years older than I. My birth was uneventful. I was very lucky as my sister's birth was complicated. She was premature and was born with complications. She has cerebral palsy and a severe hearing loss that my mother said were caused by the forceps that were used during her delivery.

My infancy was uneventful until I was about three. At that time, I accompanied my mom to the doctor for her to get a routine blood test. As the needle was stuck into her finger, I passed out cold. This was the first in a long line of fainting that are part of my life history. I can recall numerous times in elementary school when I passed out. It usually had something to do with medical situations. The mere presence of the school nurse was enough to have me flat on the floor. My head was hit so many times. I remember hitting the metal legs of the desk that were attached to the floor with bolts. It wasn't until 1985 that a diagnosis of "vasovagal syncope" was made. The diagnosis came after I had a tilt table test performed at the hospital. The doctor told me that I broke the record on the table. I passed out quicker than anyone else had done before me. I often wonder if all the head injuries I sustained have any connection with the fact that now I have PD. I can recall passing out in church on my first communion day and at the dentist office when I was there with a friend. I didn't even have an appointment. Then there was the time that I was a bridesmaid in a friend's wedding. That time I hit my head on the marble floor with such force that the sound of my head hitting the marble floor echoed so loudly throughout the church that the wedding vows were halted until I was taken care of.

As I go through my life's history trying to make some sense out of Parkinson's, it has become so apparent that my head has been subjected to too much abuse. I also wonder about stages of physical development and the role that it had in my PD story.

1) Passed out at Doctor's office.
2) Passed out at school.
3) Passed out at dentist office while friend was seeing dentist.
4) Passed out at first communion.

5) Passed out while standing up for a friend's wedding.

6) Passed out while having blood taken from an artery in wrist.

7) Passed out at church if I was fasting and if my hat was applying pressure near my temples. I was so happy when the church relaxed the fasting requirements and did away with the silly rule that women had to cover their heads.

8) Passed out when friends were discussing their medical problems.

As I was entering puberty, I experienced Grand Mal Seizures. The majority of the seizures happened while I was sleeping at night. I would know that I had had a seizure when I would wake up with blood all over my pillow and a sore tongue from where I had bitten it during the seizure. Seizures were not much of a problem after my teen years. I was on anti-seizure drugs until two years ago. I have had numerous EEG tests. Nothing abnormal ever appeared on these brain wave images.

When I was nineteen years old, my head got hit again. This time I was a passenger in a car accident. I was thrown into the steering wheel and received lacerations around my right eye and bumps and bruises on my forehead. I had a concussion. My forehead and right eye hit a plastic steering wheel knob. The impact of my head on the plastic knob caused the knob to shatter. I had to have green plastic pieces removed from my injuries before they could suture the wounds. I was left with considerable scarring. I have had reconstructive surgery twice to minimize the scars. As I have aged, the scars are more noticeable again.

I continued on with the good life. I went away to college for the last two years. I graduated from Illinois State University with a bachelor's degree in education. I started my career as a speech therapist in a public school. I remained at home with my parents during my first year of teaching.

In July 1962, I married the love of my life who has been with me during the last fifty-two years. His role has changed during the years.

He has always been a good provider and a hard worker. We worked together as a team raising our three children. Now Steve has become my care giver. He does whatever is necessary to assist me as I continue to battle with PD and the pains of a broken hip that has not gotten better with therapy, pain shots, and pills. Prior to our marriage I remember telling Steve about my seizure disorder. This was my mom's advice. She said I should make him aware of my medical problems prior to a commitment. His reaction was as I expected it would be. I was fine in his eyes. Little did any of us have any idea that Parkinson's was in my future.

The next significant blow to my head came in my mid-twenties. I had my little daughter, Katie, outside playing with her friend. They decided to play at Barbara's house. When it was time for Katie to come home, she did not respond to my asking her to come home. I attempted to jump the fence to physically bring her back home. Unfortunately, my foot caught in the fence and I landed on my chin. This blow to the chin caused another concussion. I suffered a temporary loss of vision.

Thinking back to my young adult life, I was very busy with three kids. Katie was born in October of 1964. I had a very quick delivery with no complications. In June of 1966 I gave birth to John. This, too, was a smooth, quick delivery.

My third pregnancy was not easy. I was admitted into the hospital to try to diagnose the pains I was experiencing during my last trimester. This was before ultra sounds were used with pregnant women. I was sent home on bed rest with no answers or relief for my pain. It wasn't until December 6th, 1970, two months before my due date, the cause become clear. I experienced an "abrupt placenta preview". In plain English this meant that the afterbirth came first. It can cause the baby to lose all of its nourishment if the baby is not removed quickly enough. Because of this the doctor performed an emergency Cesarean section and Mark was born. Mom and baby were both very tired. We stayed in the hospital for ten days. All is well that ends well. Mark is now a strapping young man who among other accomplishments is a volunteer fireman.

I stayed home as a full time mom until the late 1970s. It was then that I went back to work. I started slowly as a substitute teacher. I stayed in good health until 1985 when I experienced chest pains that put me in the hospital cardiac unit. It was determined that my gallbladder was the cause of the pain. I did not have gall stones but my gall bladder was not functioning correctly. After the gall bladder was surgically removed, my pains dissipated. It was during the bouts with the gall bladder that I began to pass out again as I had when I was young. We called a cardiologist in. Through a diagnostic tilt table test, he diagnosed vasovagal syncope, a condition that I have had since I was a toddler. I still have this condition but am able to recognize situations when I might have problems. I can usually avert passing out by taking precautions. I was then put on blood pressure medications. My pill list started to grow. I now had seizure medications and blood pressure medicine to take daily. At this time I had no idea that Parkinson's was in my future.

As I was growing older, I started experiencing more physical symptoms. I also began more self-diagnosis. This is easy to do when you are approaching retirement. I had more aches and pains and, of course, menopause was getting blamed for everything. If I couldn't offer a different reason for whatever I was experiencing, menopause was always a convenient excuse.

The year 2005 is very significant in my life. I was planning on retiring in June so the April spring break was going to be my last spring break. We had planned a trip to Colorado to attend the baptism of my first great niece. The plane ride was uneventful. It was great to see family, friends and the beautiful mountains. Steve and I took our rental car to Colorado Springs to see the Garden of the Gods. I didn't see much of them as I fell during our first stop. I could not get up and walk. There were lots of people present who were so helpful in getting aid for me. I was taken by ambulance to a hospital with a badly broken ankle. I often wonder if this was a fall caused by Parkinson's or if it was just a fall for no particular reason. I had plates and screws put in my ankle, missed the baptism and had to fly home with a broken ankle.

Once I got home, life became more challenging. The orthopedic doctor I saw decided I should wear a hard cast on my foot for six weeks. I had less than six weeks to go before I retired from my teaching career. I had to finish teaching, close up my two school offices, attend numerous retirement functions, etc. I did all of this from a walker or wheelchair.

That June I retired from teaching. Immediately upon retirement I started to have health problems. I had a diverticulitis attack which landed me in the hospital with emergency surgery that took nine inches of my colon and left me with a colostomy that was reversed in September. As I was recovering, I was becoming aware of the fact that my balance was being compromised. I didn't dwell on these problems as I was excited about retirement and the new avenues that were opening for me.

We moved to The Villages in June 2006. Excitement of a new world kept me busy. This was the first big move we had ever made. We had lived in our Elmhurst home for thirty-four years. We had a very busy month getting ready to relocate. I worked from sun up to sun down. I was fatigued most of the time and I attributed it to the fact that I was still recuperating from all of my medical problems. I also attributed it to aging and menopause and anything else I could conjure up. Parkinson's was certainly not in my thoughts at all. I knew next to nothing about the disease. Now I know that I had Parkinson's before I came to Florida in 2006.

I had cataract surgery in May 2007.

My Parkinson's was not diagnosed until November 2008. During the two years of not knowing what was causing my symptoms, I was having the time of my life. I enjoyed moving into a new neighborhood where everyone was new. I made friends with Alice, my neighbor. Making a new friend at this time in my life was an experience. I hope everyone can experience this. Friendships are formed at different times of your life for different reasons. It has been my good fortune to realize that friendships that are formed in the twilight years of your life are probably the most important ones of all. Alice and I hit it off immediately. We shared common interests. She liked to walk, sew, knit, shop, socialize, exercise and enjoy life to its fullest. She was also extremely caring. When I was diagnosed with Parkinson's, she encouraged me to join the support groups. To make it easier for me to attend she went with me as a support person. This worked out well for quite a while. Then, the roles started to change. Alice was slipping fast into dementia. I was becoming her support person. Alice loved everyone and provided support to anyone who needed it at the PD meetings. Alice has since gone to her reward. I miss her so much and think about her so often. She lived directly across the street from me so I continue to see her home every time I look out of my kitchen windows. Her house has been sold and the new owners have moved in. They have gone back to Michigan for the summer. They are going to be snowbirds for a while.

*****

The following is a chronological progression of my life with PD.

<u>November 2008, the beginning of Parkinson's:</u> I questioned my doctor about the following symptoms.

- Toes curl under—move involuntarily (right foot)
- Movements very slow
- Right foot drops sometimes while walking
- Posture—tendency to lean forward
- Balance getting worse

Based on the above my doctor suggested that I see a neurologist for a diagnosis. She never intimated that she thought it could be PD.

<u>November 18, saw neurologist:</u>
- Diagnosed with Parkinson's

- Put on generic form of Sinemet (Reaction: raw tongue, swollen throat)
- Put on Mirapex (Reaction: nausea making me bedridden for a day)

Stopped meds until after Christmas trip:
- Very tired during trip

December 31, started Requip XL 2 mg:
- Some mouth irritation but not too bad
- Two weeks later dosage to 4 mg – mouth still sore but not too bad
- One week later dosage to 6 mg—back to raw tongue & swollen throat

January 29, 2009:
- Dropped dosage back to 2 mg for six weeks – minimal mouth irritation

July 10, 2009, symptoms:
- Toes on right foot – curled under
- Toes on left foot moving when they are in relaxed position
- Minor tremors of fingers and hands

- Tremors of face when eating (occasional)
- Voice volume is too soft
- Swallowing is problematic (clearing food from mouth difficult)
- Eating is slow and cumbersome (appetite is small)
- Balance is poor
- Fatigue
- Slow motor movement – stop in middle of movement

Dr. Nieves prescribed Azilect—No reaction—still taking it.

Other drugs tried include:
o Sinemet – name brand
o Amantadine
o Artane
Reactions to all drugs except Azilect.

June 20, 2010, current symptoms:
- Toes curling and moving despite Botox injections

- Poor balance
- Extreme slowness in movement
- Minor tremors
- Small steps
- Small writing
- Dystonia (catchall term for unexplained movement in PD)
- Difficulty eating
- Weight loss
- Fatigue

I have become too familiar with the medical facilities and personalities of all who claim a part of my story. I established myself with a cardiologist. I am still with him. I also wanted a primary care physician, had several and am still looking for one I would like to keep. I am in the process right now of looking for a doctor who is on staff and has privileges within the Ocala hospitals.

November 2011: I fell and broke my hip. This was the worst incident that has happened to me. I still have therapy twice a week because the pain in my hip is often excruciating. I have been to many doctors and therapists to try to get some peace. They seem to agree that the orthopedic surgeon who performed the partial hip replacement left me with one leg one inch longer than the other leg. I now have a marked case of drop foot. I have to wear a brace on my right shoe and a lift in my left shoe to compensate for the short leg. This operation was performed in The Villages Regional Medical Center.

January 2012: another accident to my head

I took a ride down my driveway backwards in my walker and ended up on my back seated in the walker with my head resting on the pavement. All this happened despite the fact that two people witnessed my ride and ran to try to help me. The ride was just too quick.

October 2012: Fell in Wisconsin and fractured my pelvis and back.

I was hospitalized at the Villages with a bowel problem. Received a very expensive shot for my blocked bowel. Went into rehab. I was in rehab over the Thanksgiving holiday. I went to Premiere to see my primary doctor at the time.

December 6, 2013:
I had a weird experience. I went to lunch with friends. Had a good time, came home, was talking to my husband and then my nose started to bleed. This was the first time I ever had a nose bleed. It would not stop. Steve took me to the doctor. He could not control the bleeding with ordinary packing. He sent me to the Villages hospital where I waited hours. They put a tampon type packing in my nose to try to stop the bleeding. This was unsuccessful also. I ended up at Munroe Hospital in Ocala because they had an ENT on call. I developed toxic shock syndrome from the nose and I also had "heart involvement".

April 2014:
Hopefully the following will be my last falling incident. I got up in the morning and just fell down in my bathroom. I hit my

forehead/temple area on the right side of my head on the sink. This fall caused a large brain bleed. It left me incapacitated as I had never experienced before. My brain was hit this time with enough force to push me into dementia. I was in rehab for four weeks after the initial week at Munroe Hospital. My second brain scan indicated that the brain bleed is gone now and my brain is functioning normally again.

*****

August 2015: Well, my wish to function normally did not last long. I managed to keep up with my past pattern of falling. My next fall came in January 2015. We called 911, next stop: Munroe Hospital. The routine was the same. I had x-rays; then the doctor checked me out and read the x-rays. The results were different. This time I had broken the other hip. The left hip was a significantly different type of break. Fortunately the hip could be pinned without a replacement part.

My left hip healed and responded well to

rehab. While I was in rehab, I continued to have major difficulty with my right hip. It dislocated. The doctor snapped it back into position but the bones had other ideas. They now have dubbed my right hip "permanently disabled". What this means to me is that I cannot bear weight on my right leg. I will never be able to walk again without assistance. My wings have been clipped and my independence compromised. I am able to transfer using a wheelchair, pivoting on my left foot.

I have been in therapy since the initial hp break (November 2011). You must be diligent with therapy if you want to beat Parkinson's. I have had many different therapists in many different locations. I started with an in-patient therapy program. Then I was enrolled in the home health model. Therapists come to my home for personal therapy.

I had hoped that my days in medical facilities were over. Since the hip fracture appears to be a dead issue, I have come to terms with my disability. This past May I picked up an extremely contagious bacterial infection that required isolation for care. It's just part of the picture when you are dealing Parkinson's. I spent the entire month of June in the hospital.

I have been home more than a month now and am doing much better. Life is starting over. There are so many factors to deal with as we age. The longer we live, the more opportunities we have to smile and not dwell on the negative.

When I was asked to write this account I wasn't sure I wanted to come out to the public. After a lot of soul searching I decided to tell my story, hoping that there is something in my story that readers may find helpful.

My final thought is that PD will throw some unexpected curves. Just remember: curves go up as well as down. Life is good.

~~Ann Klonicke

Book #3

PARKINSON'S CARE GIVERS

Our

Care Givers

Are

Most

Important

You'll feel desperate ~~
      ~~but the reward is in the giving.
                                    Ed Kluft

CARE GIVERS

The Hapless Stages: Unlucky · Unhappy · Untimely

The faithful or *sometime* faithful CARE GIVER is the unsung hero of this book. I have asked the best of the ones I know to answer some questions about their experiences. I am also including my experiences as a care giver. One doesn't always receive. Occasionally one must give even in the midst of one's own need. I will just keep writing as I wait for the others' response.

1. How difficult do you find keeping work going for two?

2. How is the communication aspect of you relationship?

3. Are you able to continue being pleasant or not?

4. In your opinion will the future hold *more* promise or *less*?

****

I will say I have some good days and some really bad ones. Winter temperatures are coming. I really have to take care of myself which makes the future not so bright as I would have hoped. It's the "simple" things that make it hard. For example: putting each leg in its proper location in my long pants takes time to work out logistically. I need to wear socks and shoes, which poses a problem as well. My right leg can lift to pull a sock on, oh but I can't lift my left leg enough to get the sock over my toes. I catch my breath then stretch my toes down, heel up to pull the sock under and grab the top edge and pull the rest of the way. Yesterday, Monday, February 03, 2014, was one of my very worst. I have been having a bout with Vertigo and the pill for that is Dramamine for seasickness. Why? The house wasn't moving and I wasn't on a vessel but at least it has been working.

****

CARE GIVERS RESPOND

In the first several days many have returned. No one signed up for this job they now have because who would have thought dear ones would get sick and require the vigilance of care that that would be needed in their later years. In their marriage vows everyone agreed to: "in sickness and health till death do us part" meant with the new title, the care giver now has to do, "bathe, dress, and maintain the needed hygiene till death do us part".

****

Each of us continues with trial and error just like the renowned neurologists we go to. At their very best they prescribe for us what they think we would need and hope and wait for results. They don't call to see how we're doing. They say, instead, see me in three months. I have gotten discouraged going to my neurologist realizing if I were to contract another disease he would refer me to a specialist which could be very well be my primary care doctor.

After this awakening, on my next visit to my primary care doctor, I steered the discussion where I wanted. He said he would take over my Parkinson's case. He had me walk down the hall and back. He tested my reaction like blocking his hands as they moved toward me, same test the neurologist preformed, and sent me home. Back in four months. I'm in February.

During the wait I had a spitfire of an attack of Dyskinesia at Panera's. My entire insides went into and stayed in motion. I was asked what it felt like. I couldn't describe it—not a stomach ache or sore throat. It's everything inside me gone haywire at once.

****

Phillip & Ed Kluft (Cancer) My son Phillip, 21 years old, complained of severe headaches May, 1987. We were fortunate. The leading brain surgeon in Washington, D.C., came out of retirement to take the case. The investigative surgery produced evidence of cancer in Phillip's hypothalamus. The surgeon said if Phillip were his son, he would not pursue a remedy. Doing nothing didn't set well with me. We were able to get him into NIH (National Institute of Health) because of his age. There they did what they could to no avail. Four months later Phillip passed away. A dreadful event to lose a child at any age.

Lee Thomas & Nick Rapagna (PD) She says on a scale of 1 to 10 with 10 being the most difficult, I would rate my work load difficulty at 7. I do expect this will increase as Nick's disease progresses. Communication is difficult. I have always been a communicator, but Nick not so much, and with his speech difficulties now even less so. I find his speech impairment one of the most difficult elements of his disease to deal with to date. We are still able to be pleasant with one another. There are many times when I feel very frustrated and even angry that this disease has changed our life together so much. But then I think how much more it has taken away from him and how positive he remains in spite of it. I have tremendous admiration and love for my husband. Lee is a real giving Care giver for Nick who at this moment is taking care of Lee.

Helene & Ed Zeigler (PD) In a very brief message: Helene has no problem doing work for two. Ed does have a hearing issue along with his Parkinson's and she says they are pleasant with each other.

Ellen & Melvyn Pell (PD) Ellen writes her care giver's perspective: Melvin is easy to deal with today. We are still able to be very pleasant with one another. There are many times when I feel truly frustrated and even angry that this disease has changed OUR life together so much. But then I think how much more it has taken away from him and how positive he remains in spite of it. I have tremendous admiration and love for my husband. I depended on him constantly. I would say things three or more times. I try to be pleasant because Mel cannot help being so sick. It's very hard and I find myself losing patience. I am dedicated to his wellbeing and will continue to be the best I can be. Ellen is a genuine care giver making Mel a lucky person

Ellen does have one other care giving obligation: her sister, who has been in an institution eight years. Ellen is her only family now. Before the sister was institutionalized the family tried having her in her own apartment. They were told she would have to leave because she was urinating on the lobby furniture. She is apt to urinate wherever she might be—in a taxi or a doctor's office. It's an embarrassment wherever she goes. She has multiple problems. Among them is Turner Syndrome, a genetic disorder found in women causing small stature. She also has OCD, Obsessive Compulsive Disorder, and Schizophrenia. She's 62 now and very child-like. The problems will not be solved. Ellen remains the care giver for her only sibling and the only family left for her.

Sheila Feige (PD) who suggested the subtitle: "Life is what happens when you have other Plans". How intuitive this title, how generous this good person. For that reason she has shared with us how she juggles the need when she has both roles of having Parkinson's and being a care giver when necessary for her husband Gary. When he's under the weather with a cold or when he's having foot surgery, anything can keep him off his feet and Sheila on hers. Her answer: "I love how he takes care of me and I enjoy when I can care for him". Sheila is a very sincere person and is true in her efforts.

Phil & Nancy Matis (PD) Phil says it is not hard to do work around the house. Nancy helps me to do the work that she can and then tells me what still needs to be done. I appreciate her telling me what to do. We need to check our schedules to take her to doctors and do some of the food shopping. I am a quiet person and as a result do not communicate my feelings very well to Nancy. We are now working to help improve what I need to help her better. I want to be pleasant with my wife no matter what comes down the line in the future. We must accept whatever comes to us and talk about it and then make a decision together for what will be best for her. If we work together and communicate together during our lives we will be able to accept whatever comes out way. We have accepted it before. We need to continue this open dialog so we can both be happy with the decisions we make. This is a real couple that I enjoy being with at the Fight Club exercising as we do as a group.

Georgia & Darrell Emge (PD) It is becoming more and more difficult. Everywhere I look, inside and out, there's work that needs some tending to. If we have a bad night that is not restful, the next day we both need naps. Darrell doesn't want me to doing all the work and says we should hire someone to do it. I feel guilty spending money on that when I am capable of doing most of the chores. The neurologist said for him to give so much up. He has a lot going wrong at the same time. Since retiring and moving to The Villages, the first two years were the best and last five years have gone downhill quickly. I blame back surgery in 2009 and the anesthesia and pain meds causing the beginning of his dementia. That's when the hallucinations began. This left for a year or so and returned two years later and remains today.

Our relationship is not as good as it used to be. His dementia (short term memory) causes him to forget things very quickly. He wants to always be right. When we are trying to socialize he is very impatient when I'm talking to people and wants to leave. Of course so far I'm able to continue being his care giver which at times can be unpleasant I must admit. Thank God we still have many good times. If my health would fail, God forbid, it would be disastrous. He could not carry on very well on his own. His health issues have grown too severe.

Darrell hasn't driven the car for two years and gave up driving the cart over a year ago. His macular degeneration is another rea- son for that. He is more comfortable with my driving but won't let me take us on a long vacation. He worries we'll get lost. We are basically joined at the hip these days. I hate to leave him alone for too long.

Anonymous Responder (PD) My husband was diagnosed about 3 years ago and I realized he needed help two years ago. He has developed into requiring constant help as his disease progresses. Because of this I have hired help for both of our chores. His deformity and the volume of his voice has reduced and due to the deformity he talks to the floor. I can only be pleasant some of the time. We have our problems mainly because he is frustrated not being able to do what he has always done and that in turn frustrates me. All in all I think I handle my new position fairly well even though I get discouraged along with him. From appearances he is getting very good help.

Pam & Shea Eaddy (PD) Pam answered the questions in the order of my request.

The most difficult time was when he was diagnosed.

Our communications are challenging at times.

Because of our communication problem being challenging at times my patience runs thin.

He is still enjoying bowling twice a week and going fishing with his buddies

Because of our strong faith in God being pleasant is in our nature. Without God being in our lives I'm not so sure of that. He is still enjoying bowling twice a week and going fishing with his buddies. Shea is in the very early stages of PD and with their faith and exercise he might delay the worst for now.

Sanford, Beverly Cohen & Me (PD) We took care of our mother until she died of natural causes at 91. She had Dementia into Alzheimer's the last two years. Our dad passed at 53 in the course of having a heart attack. He died the same night as the attack. My self-imposed challenge was to live as long as dad. I succeeded and I'm 25 years past his age. We were fortunate having grown up in a functioning family with pleasant surroundings and full time help in the house. Our mother at 85 had a triple by-pass and two years later required a double mastectomy following that two weeks later she was out playing cards with the, we call them, girls, that she went through school with. After surgery she didn't require much in the way of Caregiving. It all began after I moved to Connecticut in 1995. A year after moving to Connecticut we decided to take her car which I took up to Connecticut and sold it to one of my employees. She worried how she would get to the beauty parlor and that's when my sister came in the real Caregiving role. Her husband Sandy even more picked mom up almost daily to see to her needs and be company for her. After a great home outfitted for 6 residents was found in a very convenient in location. She enjoyed her stay there until cancer forced her to go to a hospital and shortly passed away quietly. It was in her nature to go quietly.

Sharon and Brad Clough (PD) Brad was diagnosed 3½ years ago and there was very little change in him. Mostly all I see is a tremor in his right hand and his voice is not always as strong as it once was. He does work at trying to talk louder. He keeps his physical fitness up by playing golf 2 to 3 times a week and playing Pickle Ball, plays tennis and rides his bike. He exercises to music to stimulate his brain which is important. Attending the support group three times a week is also important. If you watch him, you would not suspect he has the Parkinson's disease. Our life so far is as it always has been. I encourage him to keep active to keep the disease at bay.

Dee & Dave Jonas (PD) Dave was diagnosed 2007. It was several years before I felt that the Parkinson's diagnosis began to affect our daily lives. Turning over home care has been a gradual thing as some days are good and the tremor isn't bad, other days it is more difficult. We still share many home care responsibilities, except that we handle them differently. Some tasks are more difficult for my husband to do as the disease has progressed, but he still can do many things. I used to do all of the laundry, cooking, and cleaning but now he does more home chores to free me up to do other things that are difficult for him to do. Not being rested affects the ability to function also.

We are in our seventh year of diagnosis.

My husband has difficulty in executive functioning tasks, which includes multitasking. I think that he may always have had this challenge, but it has been exacerbated by Parkinson's. When he eats, he seems to concentrate on just eating, so conversation during meals has decreased. One of the most difficult areas to address for us was driving. At first there was a feeling of not feeling safe as we would meander over the centerline and off the road. Just about the time that I would fall asleep in the car as a passenger, we would go off the road and I would become startled. Giving up our independence is challenging for both parties involved, but important to work through for safety. As a result, I now do most of the driving and yet he still participates in driving in areas that are not congested and on roads where a lot of multi- tasking isn't as much of an issue as driving in heavy city traffic.

In the past year, I have taken on the responsibility of dividing up his pills and reminding him to take them. His tremor has affected his ability to put the small pills in the right compartment. I would find them on the floor or too many pills in one compartment. Remembering to take his medicine in a timely manner and according to instructions has been difficult.

If I were a single person, I would have most of the chores to do anyway. However, there is also a task that a care giver takes on and that is thinking for another person besides herself. I do a lot of reminding which can be a challenge. Have you taken your medicine? Have you done your exercises? Have you scheduled your appointment for …? Remembering becomes an issue and so the follow-up a care giver needs to do to stay on top of things can be very tiresome.

Sometimes it requires real honesty to let one another know how you are feeling. It requires hanging in there to resolve issues. It is important not to bottle those feelings up or they can become explosive. I don't think that my husband realizes how quiet he becomes at times, especially when he is tired and kind of zones out. In group discussion he can become very quiet, almost appearing as though he is disinterested in a conversation. Entertaining can become challenging when you need to depend on your spouse to carry the conversation while you are tending to the cooking. His taking a nap before company arrives helps with this.

We have a saying inscribed on our kitchen wall that says, "Life is not about waiting for the Storm to Pass, but learning how to Dance in the Rain!" Life on this earth was never meant to be perfect, but the attitude with which we embrace situations is so important. Parkinson's is a disease that we are living with, but it doesn't define who we are. When we are living with a disease, it important to continue creating time for things that feeds our soul, so that we can continue to give to one an- other. We are blessed and supported by family and friends alike and need to allow ourselves to be supported as well as the de- sire to support others. Our faith also supports and strengthens us. No matter how difficult we may think things are, when we focus on other's needs, our own seems to diminish. All reasons to keep us smiling!

****

This is a departure from care giving for Parkinson's. Nonetheless, it relates a very real need at a critical time for a care giver to be with a patient.

I was living temporarily with my parents in Milford and commuting to work in New York City for Martha Stewart Living Magazine. The average peak time trip door to door was approximately 2 hours each way. So needless to say getting to work or getting home I was never really able to be in a hurry.

While I was well aware that my dad had an accident on I-95, all seemed to check out and be "OK" after he went to the hospital. As usual it was downplayed by my dad on every lev- el. Even the stories of him getting lost while driving a few times weeks after were attributed to age, being tired or simply just not paying attention.

One late morning a month or so after the

accident, I received a phone call at work from my mother telling me that Dad went for a follow up doctor's appointment and after a CT scan they immediately rushed him to the hospital as they saw bleeding in his brain. Not an easy call to take and certainly not ideal when it takes 2 hours to get home. Of course, I left right away and met my mother and father at the hospital ASAP.

After further tests, etc., it was determined that surgery was going to have to be done right away to stop the bleeding and relieve any pressure that had built up. There was no question in any of our minds as to what needed to be done.

We knew the surgery and recovery was going to be very long, so the surgeon had said to my mother and I that we should go home, eat, change and come back a bit later that night. We figured that would be best and we went home to regroup.

When the surgery was wrapping up, we received a call that we could come back to see my father. So we rushed out the door and were on our way to St. Vincent's Hospital. As a strange side note I had always worn my seatbelt in the car and my mother began wearing hers to since my father's accident, but we both had so much on our minds that we forgot. As soon as we pulled onto the exit of 95 heading south to the hospital, as luck would have it, there was a seatbelt checkpoint. Inexplicably, neither one of us had our belt on. Luckily the trooper could see the concern in our eyes and believed our story and let us go with a warning.

I remember seeing my father in the recovery room, his head wrapped up like a mummy. He wasn't able to speak but he kept reaching up to his head indicating he was in a lot of pain. We were told all went very, very well by the surgeon and we were very lucky they caught this in time. We were still concerned, but certainly relieved.

Although I don't remember the exact time frame, I do remember that the next couple days my father was progressing fabulously. His pain was subsiding, he was eating, walking and doing beautifully while recovering in the ICU.

He had to be in ICU due to the nature of the surgery and not due to any complications at that time.

One night, it was my mother, father and I visiting with each other. My father was still doing better and better. He was sitting in a visitor chair as were my mother and I. I remember to this day that he was telling funny stories about his gambling experiences all of which I had probably heard before, but they were always funny to hear. Even more so that night. During one of the stories, he was talking and all of a sudden his words of humor turned into "da, dah, dahh, dahh, dahh". My first thought was that he was being a jokester. Then his speech was again coherent but only to immediately repeat the "da, dah, dahh, dahh" except this time his facial expression was completely blank. It was at that point we knew something terrible was wrong and I ran to the nurses' station to get help.

Things became a whirlwind of confusion at that point. While at first we were told that he was having a minor seizure, not to worry;

we were then being told that his brain was "angry" and swelling. Angry was always how the surgeon explained it. It painted the perfect picture for us to understand.

Over the next few days it was a constant rotation of CT Scan, diagnosis, discussion, surgery and recovery. This seemed to repeat itself at least 100 times, although in reality it was probably only a few times at most. While initially he was "somewhat" conscious for the hours/days after the first seizure, he certainly was not in the sense of having conversations like the ones a couple nights before; however, he was responsive to some things that were being done to him and to pain. But really he was more just a living being that didn't have any intellectual capacity. To add even more bad luck to an already terrible situation, during one of his seizures while lying in bed, somehow he managed thrash around just enough to fling himself out of his bed and, of course, hitting his head on the rock solid hospital floor. We found him lying on the ground and as you may guess what followed ... CT Scan, surgery, recovery.

I can't be certain as to which surgery was the last one he had, or the last one he came back from and still had any signs of true life (other than a pulse and oxygen monitor). I do know that after one several surgeries to relieve the swelling and his angry brain, he came back into the ICU room to not wake up again and to be in a complete coma. It was really a surreal experience. There were so many ups and downs of emotions getting to that point that it was hard remember exactly how we got there.

While I was doing the best that I could to go into work in NYC in the morning, it was most important that I got back and to the hospital by early afternoon to be with my father and family. My mom had so much worry and pain in her face. She was completely overrun with devastation and fear. I can't help but think back that as few of times I lived with my parents after college, I thank God that this was one of those times. Being there at night for my mother after long days of the hospital was critical. We both need so much support and we truly leaned on each other during this time.

I was trying to be as strong as I could for her … but I guess that is all relative.

My father's coma seemed to last years. I am not even 100% positive how long it truly lasted for, I do know if was very long. I was weeks. There was nothing but beeping monitors, feeding tubes, nurses knuckling his chest or squeezing his toes to cause pain and see if he would respond. Nothing. There was even talk of how his muscles were slowly pulling him into more and more of a fetal position, as it happens when one is slipping deeper and deeper towards "the light". However, I can honestly say that despite all the worry, concern and acknowledgement of the looming possibility, I had never really thought there would be a point that a decision would ever have to be made. Maybe ignorantly so, I just thought that nature would decide that if or even when it decided to. That is until late one night when my mother and I were leaving the hospital after another long and difficult day.

The vision in my memory was that my

mom and I were leaving and were actually walking out of the elevator and into the main lobby of the hospital. By chance we had bumped into my father's main neurosurgeon's partner. I don't remember his name and only remember he was an Asian man. I had seen him many times before as when Dr. Mince was not on duty, his partner would check in on my father's progress. Well anyway, this time we were leaving and as we saw him, we stopped just to say a quick hello. He did the same. After a brief conversation of "pleasantries," if you can call it that, he turned much more serious and matter of fact. His exact words escape me today, but he stated that even if my dad were to come out of his coma, he would be a vegetable. So while keeping him alive was typical human nature, we should think about whose benefit we were keeping him alive for. We needed to think of the merciful thing to do for my father and not the selfish thing to do by keeping him lying there; to let him go in peace.

As I said earlier, this decision process had not crossed my mind at all. I don't know if it had crossed my mother's mind before this meeting with the surgeon in the lobby, but if she had thought of it, I never knew it. All of a sudden my father's coma had gone from a difficult and painful situation for all of us to an impossible an inhumane decision permeating our entire reality. Completely crushed, drove home that night not knowing what to make of everything.

Now, as my dad would describe things if you were to ask him today (or at times even if you didn't ask him) my sister and I immediately said to my mother to "ok, then just pull the plug," almost like "oh well, ho hum". And that my mother essentially fought us on this and fought to keep my father alive against my will and my sister's wishes. To set the record straight, NOTHING could be farther from the truth. My mother, sister and I were consumed by the conversation. All the reasons why she shouldn't consider letting him go, and the one and only reason why it would make sense to...for his mercy and what he would want.

Would he want to be unable to live a normal life and would he want to be a "burden" on my mother. The conversation went on and on and on. Nobody should ever have to have that conversation about a loved one. It's just not fair.

I will fully admit that I took the surgeon's point more deeply than my mother. He is smarter than me and should obviously know much more about this stuff than we would. Of course he is my dad and of course I love him for the great dad that he is/was. But my mother's love for a husband thankfully shielded her from the science of the matter and shielded her from the fact that my dad wouldn't want to be a burden on her. As a loving wife, she didn't care about what form she would have him in, she just didn't want to lose him. While her pain and grief of seeing my dad laying there in a coma was overwhelming, my mother simply wasn't ready to make that ultimate decision. She knew she was going to have to decide one day soon, she just wasn't ready that day or the next day. She needed more and pray time to hope.

While we all were hoping and praying over the next day or two at the most, the unbelievable, unexpected miracle happened and my dad began to slowly show signs of coming out of the coma and then ultimately doing so. Just a couple extra days of hoping and praying proved to be all the difference of my dad being alive today.

To this day the words of his primary surgeon Dr. Mince give me goose bumps. When he commented on my father's coming out of the coma. At my father's bedside he turned to my mother and I said "this had nothing to with science or medicine, this was something much greater than that."

****

SUMMATION OF THE BEST CARE GIVERS

I have taken this opportunity to voice my opinion on these care givers whom I have known for a while. To quote from a source: The role of a care giver is usually one that a person must take on without any prior warning. It is a major change to anyone's lifestyle. A care giver must be on-call twenty-four hours a day. They must always be on their toes. They must organize, be well informed and watchful. They must be very patient, helpful and warm-hearted towards their mate or charge's changing physical and mental condition. They must possess a determination to carefully balance the new demands that lie ahead. This is difficult to master. It's important that all care givers have inner strength and understand that this disease affects different people in different ways. In other words, the symptoms won't always be the same in all those with the disease. We already know most experience loss of smell, some tremors, deterioration of handwriting, less volume in speaking and slowness in walking.

The best of the care givers become well informed through searching answers through others in support groups. Here in The Villages that becomes easier because there so many Parkinson's sufferers and their care givers. I'm sensitive to them and their efforts because I don't have a care giver in the person I share a house with. I'm told I'm lazy. The way I usually feel, perhaps I am. The feeling discourages wanting to do chores. There's definitely a change in the person that's suffering the illness.

There is an extensive support network available. Parkinson's is very manageable through the prescription meds and exercise programs available now. It's a daily effort to see results that must be kept up. It, too, is important for the Care giver to keep up the social activities to balance their own needs. If possible, and can be afforded, getting help to come in on an agreed schedule is a great help. The role of a care giver is usually one that a person must take on without any prior warning, and yet must, to the best of their ability be ready, tackle willingly and pleasantly. Be patient, helpful, warm and watchful as the need arises. Changes can be abrupt and you must be prepared for the moments need.

Since there is such a wide variety of

symptoms, assistance should not be assumed to be the same all the time. It bears repeating, read more below.

A bit more explanation into what it really takes to be the care giver knowing it is not easy to accept first the diagnosis of the disease and then knowing it progresses as the time goes on. It's a subtle disease in the beginning. You won't know it's coming on. What should you notice? Often the first symptom is loss of the ability to smell or you may notice tremors. Personality may tone down and experience small bouts with depression. In addition, your loved one may have muscle stiffness and slowness in movements. Though these could be common problems, not all PD patients will experience them.

The most effective care giver has done the research and has learned what to do. There are support groups wherever you might be. Also, please be sure to keep others up on what you are doing. Share what you learn. Stay strong.

###